Praise for
Anxiety-Free with Food

*"If you are trying to avoid stress, you were born in the wrong era!
Liana's recipes are packed with antioxidants, magnesium, and
good healthy omega fats to help reduce stress and defeat anxiety."*
— Mark Hyman, M.D., *New York Times* best-selling
author of *Food: What the Heck Should I Eat?*

*"Anxiety-Free with Food shows us which foods to eat to support
healthy brain function and encourage positive thinking. Anxiety is often
associated with low levels of nutrients; focusing on the foods from this
book will support you with magnesium and omega-3, two important
elements for soothing nerves. Doing things that are pleasurable, including
eating wholesome nourishing foods, is the quickest way to increase your
levels of important neurotransmitters such as serotonin and dopamine. This
book offers easy tips for enhancing your nutrition and plenty of recipes that
can instantly boost your feel-good hormones. Liana reminds you that
life is not about striving for perfection and encourages you to do
what you can and nourish your body a little at a time."*
— Christiane Northrup, M.D., *New York Times* best-selling
author of *Women's Bodies, Women's Wisdom*

*"Few of us realize how the foods we eat can directly affect our moods—
both positively and negatively! Scientific research has demonstrated that
there is a link between nutrition and anxiety.* Anxiety-Free with Food
*shows you which foods and supplements can help put you in a better state
of mind. Liana's recipes are rich in B vitamins, vitamin D, magnesium,
protein, probiotics, healthy fats, and other essential nutrients to support
your mental health as well as decrease inflammation. When you get this
book, you'll be doing your body and mind a favor."*
— Dr. Josh Axe, DNM, DC, CNS, doctor of natural
medicine, founder of DrAxe.com

"Using the concept of the 7 Toxicities as one of the key pillars in our philosophy at the Centers for Advanced Medicine, we have now treated patients from 93 different countries for the most serious of medical conditions, including late-stage cancer, heart disease, stroke, and more. The theory and postulate have now been tested and proven and are the underlying fundamental basis of how we approach treatment of all chronic disease in our clinics. So what's all this got to do with anxiety and how is it relevant to this book? Well, the answer may very well be the aha moment our planet needs today more than ever!

"Even though no one of the 7 Toxicities is more important than the other, special acknowledgment ought to be given to the 5th Toxicity. The 5th Toxicity is the emotional/psychological toxicity that, at some level, affects every single person and perhaps all life-forms on this planet. It is this emotional/ psychological toxicity that contributes and ignites the fires of chronic disease and fuels it to progress rampantly . . . in many cases, insidiously. And the manifestation of that progression takes the form of anxiety, leading to fear and depression, progressing to hopelessness and worse.

"Liana Werner-Gray's book Anxiety-Free with Food is a great place to begin to learn how we can help our physiology achieve a better foundation to help tolerate the bombardment of the inevitable baggage we accumulate. The accumulation of the traumas we experience as we grow and mature, along with their impact on our physiology, has been virtually ignored. In fact, in my professional opinion, it has become the most insidious causation of pathology playing a leading role in all chronic disease. This may at first seem like another over-the-top statement. However, the more chronically ill patients I see, the clearer it becomes to me that if the emotional/psychological underlying issues are not addressed adequately to resolve anxiety and fear, the patient will never recover and regain their health. Resolving conflict, alleviating anxiety, and focusing on love are the most important things we as a society must realize in order to evolve and survive on our planet. Liana does an outstanding job in giving us the first place to start in this journey by helping us improve our physiology with the right foods to help us become anxiety-free!"

— Rashid A. Buttar, D.O., FAAPM, FACAM, FAAIM, medical director for the Centers for Advanced Medicine and Clinical Research

ANXIETY
FREE
WITH
FOOD

ALSO BY
LIANA WERNER-GRAY

Cancer-Free with Food: A Step-by-Step Plan
with 100+ Recipes to Fight Disease, Nourish
Your Body & Restore Your Health

The Earth Diet: Your Complete Guide
to Living Using Earth's Natural Ingredients

All of the above are available at your local
bookstore, or may be ordered by visiting:

Hay House USA: www.hayhouse.com®
Hay House Australia: www.hayhouse.com.au
Hay House UK: www.hayhouse.co.uk
Hay House India: www.hayhouse.co.in

ANXIETY FREE

WITH

FOOD

NATURAL, SCIENCE-BACKED STRATEGIES TO RELIEVE STRESS AND SUPPORT YOUR MENTAL HEALTH

LIANA WERNER-GRAY

HAY HOUSE, INC.
Carlsbad, California • New York City
London • Sydney • New Delhi

Published in the United States by: Hay House, Inc.: www.hayhouse.com®
Published in Australia by: Hay House Australia Pty. Ltd.: www.hayhouse.com.au
Published in the United Kingdom by: Hay House UK, Ltd.: www.hayhouse.co.uk
Published in India by: Hay House Publishers India: www.hayhouse.co.in

Indexer: Beverlee Day
Cover and interior design: Julie Davison

Library of Congress Cataloging-in-Publication Data

Names: Werner-Gray, Liana, 1987- author.
Title: Anxiety-free with food : natural, science-backed strategies to
   relieve stress and support your mental health / Liana Werner-Gray.
Description: 1st edition. | Carlsbad, California : Hay House, Inc., [2020]
Identifiers: LCCN 2020039174 | ISBN 9781401961763 (trade paperback) | ISBN
   9781401961749 (ebook)
Subjects: LCSH: Anxiety--Alternative treatment. | Natural
   foods--Therapeutic use. | Cooking (Natural foods) | Self-care, Health.
Classification: LCC RC531 .W434 2020 | DDC 616.85/220654--dc23
LC record available at https://lccn.loc.gov/2020039174

Tradepaper ISBN: 978-1-4019-6176-3
E-book ISBN: 978-1-4019-6174-9
Audiobook ISBN: 978-1-4019-6175-6

11 10 9 8 7 6 5 4 3 2
1st edition, December 2020

Printed in the United States of America

To everyone who has been
affected by anxiety and wants
to enjoy a good life.

CONTENTS

INTRODUCTION

Life is good and meant to be enjoyed. If you aren't there yet, you can get there. Living in this day and age is tough—it's not easy for anyone. Dr. Mark Hyman says if you are trying to avoid stress, you were born in the wrong era. There are countless stressful situations to confront, big and small, every day, and coping is so much harder when we feel anxious. Anxiety plagues millions of people around the world. Along with depression, it is estimated to affect at least 55 million people in the United States alone.[1] Roughly 18 percent of the population has mild, moderate, or severe symptoms of anxiety in a given year.[2]

I was once part of this statistic. By my late teens, I felt anxious—looking back, it was likely the result of issues with my family and graduating high school while not knowing what would come next. I was just living and breathing and doing my best to function. For many years, I thought I might be "stuck" like that forever and would just have to accept that life was hard and painful, and every day felt like a repetitive nightmare of self-doubt and anxiety.

When I was 26 years old, I was diagnosed with severe anxiety and depression by a psychiatrist. The doctor offered me a prescription for medication, but although I was in deep emotional pain, I had a wrenching feeling that if I were to take a drug it would only make matters worse. I believed medication would so numb my pain that it would hinder me from doing deep inner healing work to set me free from this debilitating disorder for the rest of my life.

Please know that I do not discredit the value of modern medicine—many people with depression and anxiety do very well on medication. A functional-medicine approach might include addressing lifestyle choices along with taking medications. But I didn't think taking pharmaceuticals was the right path for me. I remember thinking, *I want to get to the root cause. Why do I have depression? Why do I have anxiety? What can I do about it other than being on medication my entire life?* I was confident that diet would play a role in it.

GROWING UP IN AUSTRALIA

I've always been interested in doing the inner work, and perhaps this is because of my upbringing.

When I was a child, my father was living off the land in a small town outside of Perth, where he grew his own food, made his own wine, and painted. He used the vegetables from his garden in his restaurant and sold his paintings there. There was no TV or radio at his place, and when my sisters and I would visit, we were told to use water sparingly as it was pumped straight from a well; he wasn't connected to the town's water source. He was an ultimate naturalist, and I respect that about him.

My parents split when I was three years old, at which point my mum moved us to Alice Springs, which is smack-bang in the middle of Australia—total Outback Australia. This is where I spent most of my upbringing. My mother was a beautiful minimalist when it came to her cooking, wardrobe, and home. Our house and lifestyle were so simple.

The community and landscape in Alice Springs shape my life even as it is now. At my school, half of the kids were white like me, and half were Aborigines. We were taught about Aboriginal history and other indigenous cultures growing up. Our school often took us out on excursions to teach us Aboriginal ways; they showed us "bush tucker," which is food that comes straight from the bush, and how to survive off the land. As I grew older, I gained even more respect for the wisdom of the indigenous people in how they lived off the land for centuries. They didn't have many of today's diseases because they didn't have any processed foods full of additives and preservatives, weird fillers, and artificial sweeteners to mess with their body's natural harmony.

My close friends among the indigenous people in our area taught me that healing *anything* was possible. Note that healing was never guaranteed—but it was *possible*. They addressed things like wounds, snakebites, and illnesses using the resources they had available to them (they called it bush medicine) and praying with their tribe. The tribe would get together and sing out to spirit to invite healing, and it worked. The lesson here is that the path to wellness is one we don't need to face alone. Just as the tribe comes together to offer support to a member, we would rely on our own family, friends, trusted health professionals, and other experts for support, wisdom, and advice.

As a result of my upbringing, I always have believed that no matter what issue we are faced with, we have a chance of healing it. This is why, when I was diagnosed with anxiety and depression—a condition that I had never had a name for until then and just assumed was normal—I knew deep down that I would not accept living with it for the rest of my life. Once it was out in the open, I took it on.

Experiencing Healing Firsthand

There was another reason I believed in my power to heal. A few years prior to my diagnosis of depression and anxiety, I'd contended successfully with a different health challenge. When I was 21, a biopsy of my throat revealed I had a 3.7–centimeter mass in my throat. A golf-ball-size lump popped out one day without warning and turned out to be an early-stage cancer. For half a decade, I had been binge-eating junk food—my "drug" of choice to soothe my anxiety—and it had destroyed my health.

By the time I was 16, I was already addicted to sugary processed foods. Even though I knew that eating foods straight from nature would give me the health I wanted, I just couldn't do it. The addictive cravings I felt were stronger than my ability to resist them, and my emotional pain was so intense that as soon as I felt a flutter of nerves, I would run to food to get a five-minute "high." In a typical day, I would eat gummy bears for breakfast, an entire block of chocolate and packet of cookies for a snack, and fast food for lunch and dinner. I rarely gave my body any wholesome nutrients from vegetables and fruits. I believe that because I deprived my body of nourishment for so many years, eventually my lymphatic system became so clogged with junk that it could no longer remove toxins and formed the mass in my neck.

The diagnosis of cancer was the painful wake-up call that I needed to clean up my habits. Thankfully, because of my upbringing, I believed I could use food to improve my condition. I started juicing and detoxing my body, inventing recipes to feed my cravings using wholesome, natural ingredients. I had stumbled upon a strategy known as *replacement therapy*. When I had a craving for French fries, for example, I made some by chopping potatoes and frying them in olive oil or baking them in the oven. (I have since changed my frying oil to coconut oil because of the higher smoke point—the temperature at which an oil begins to smoke and oxidize.)

I also developed wholesome versions of recipes for chicken nuggets, cookie dough, chocolate balls . . . and the list goes on and on. Soon I stopped craving unhealthy foods altogether and started to crave the recipes I was making instead.

Today I call this approach the Food Upgrade System. Chapter 5 of this book is dedicated to feeding you healthful versions of all the things you may crave when you feel anxious.

Within three months of eating in this new way, the tumor in my throat had entirely dissolved. I felt so passionate about sharing with the world what I was doing and the success I was having with my recipes that I created the *Earth Diet* blog. This turned into my first published book! It became my life purpose and mission to help other people heal with food.

ADDRESSING MY ANXIETY HEAD-ON

Better health, a popular blog, and a best-selling book?! I had it all and should have been on top of the world. To be honest, some days I was flying high emotionally. But I still could be triggered emotionally and find myself in the midst of a panic attack with racing heart and breathing troubles. There were days when I was meant to attend events and scheduled work, but I felt so anxious I stayed in bed terrified of getting up and having to face the world, and at the same time terrified of staying in bed. It felt like nothing I did could allow me escape from the doom and gloom of anxiety and the ever-present fear of a bad future.

One morning, while sitting at home and sipping a cup of tea, I realized that I felt empty inside. It suddenly occurred to me that I had a bigger responsibility now that my dream was a reality: I had written a book and needed to be held accountable at a higher level. I made an appointment to speak with a psychiatrist on the recommendation of a good friend, which was how I got my diagnosis of anxiety and depression. That's when I was faced with a prescription and a decision to make.

Before taking medication for anxiety, I thought, *Let me try and address it with food.* But how?

The first thing I did was to research anxiety. What is it, and where does it come from? Does anxiety come from the mind, from thoughts affecting the body? Or does it come from a problem in the body that agitates the nervous system and throws it out of whack?

Maybe it went as far back as childhood—was it a side effect of being a child whose parents split? Sometimes I felt inner turmoil because my mom was having health challenges. Whatever the reason, I was ready to understand it so I could address the nutritional aspects underlying it.

UNDERSTANDING THE NUTRITIONAL FACTORS OF ANXIETY

The main dietary issues people with anxiety are facing, I discovered, are likely to be deficiencies in omega-3 fatty acids, magnesium, and amino acids. Without these, your brain won't function optimally, and you'll soon begin displaying some symptoms of anxiety—and also depression—everything from irritability and mood swings to insomnia, digestive upset, and a sense of impending doom.[3]

I got a blood test done and asked my doctor to check if my omega-3 count was low. Sure enough, I was deficient in fatty acids! The doctor recommended I take fish oil supplements right away. A few days later, I felt better and was sure the fish oil supplements had taken effect. I also started to incorporate more omega-3 fats in my meals, using ingredients like salmon, chia seeds, hempseeds, coconut oil, olive oil, walnuts, and avocado.

Also, I dove into researching the role of the nervous system: the brain, spinal cord, and nerves. This is the body's communication system, which controls much of what your body does. It allows us to do things like walk, speak, swallow, breathe, and learn, and controls how our bodies react in an emergency. I learned that the nervous system can be damaged by diseases; injuries (trauma), especially to the head and spinal cord; blood supply problems (vascular disorders); and mental health problems, such as anxiety disorders, depression, or psychosis.[4]

Guess what: Another disorder of the nervous system is a tumor! Perhaps I had done damage to my nervous system early on when I polluted my body with junk foods? It struck me that—wow—I could still have some damage in my nervous system although my tumor was fully healed. Again, I did my nutritional research and then incorporated foods into my diet to address it. In my case, I used chocolate in its raw form (cacao) and chlorophyll in green juices and liquid supplements. Boy, did I eat a lot of chocolate!

My research also led me to understand that another factor causing anxiety is inflammation.[5] This was fascinating because I already knew that inflammation causes weight gain and difficulty losing weight, arthritis, all major degenerative diseases, including heart disease, cancer, hypertension, and diabetes, fever, chills, loss of energy, mood swings, headaches, stiffness, and fatigue. I just did not know that inflammation was a cause of anxiety!

This was great news because the diet I ate to heal my tumor was loaded with antioxidant fruits and vegetables. I focused on eating as many servings of vegetables and salads in a day as possible, at least once a day, and I could definitely feel a difference in my body and mind.

I hope it excites you to discover that there is much hope for people suffering today. There is a lot of science that explains why certain foods may reduce stress and anxiety. Knowing this should give you confidence and empower you.

THE PROMISE OF A BRIGHT FUTURE AHEAD

Fast-forward several years. I now know for certain that life *is* good and meant to be enjoyed, even though we are living in a historical era of great difficulties—military conflicts overseas, a downward-spiraling economy, climate changes, a global pandemic, and societal and cultural upheaval that feels like a war. For many of us, the big battle is the one happening in our hearts, minds, and bodies. But no matter what else is going on outside us, inside we can feel unwavering contentment and joy. At the very least, each of us can enjoy peace of mind and peace within our physical body because of *knowing* that it is being taken care of the best it possibly can be through high-quality foods and excellent nutrition. Our physical bodies respond so positively to the natural chemistry of the healthy foods we put into them.

According to the National Institute of Mental Health, anxiety disorders are the most common mental health concern in the United States. Yet many people are keeping their feelings a secret and suffering silently. For a while, I did the same, trying to project that I had everything under control. Our society puts pressure on us to keep up appearances. The bigger problem, in my opinion, is that people don't know how closely tied to nutrition anxiety is, so they miss an opportunity to heal.

Of course the cause of your anxiety could lie deeper, perhaps in wounds from childhood or traumatic events. If you feel like your anxiety is rooted in your heart and mind, I can relate. Please consider psychological counseling; in the meantime, the foods and supplements I describe here may still help your situation. I also offer some techniques for soothing the mind, soul, heart, and emotions on my website that may be helpful to you: LianaWernerGray.com/AnxietyFree.

It's been eight years since I was diagnosed with severe anxiety and depression, and I am so happy to report that I do not suffer as severely anymore. I do sometimes experience mild depression and anxiety; after all, recovery is a process, not a single event. I get blood work done every year or two to check that my vitamin levels are sufficient, which is how I can be so sure that my anxiety and depression aren't related to a lack of the right nutrients. I feel free and I am excited about the future, whereas before I used to dread it. This is common for people who suffer with anxiety and depression because we get stuck in thinking, *It is always going to be like this, and I don't want to have to experience that for an entire lifetime!*

There are many approaches that can contribute to easing your anxiety, including positive thinking, emotional healing, spiritual awakening, behavioral therapy, psychoanalysis, and pharmaceutical medications. The scope of this book, however, does not include *all* the therapies for anxiety, so I urge you to research any therapies that you feel may be helpful to you. Even if you're not certain that your anxiety is tied to your diet, I encourage you to just try the foods and dietary plan in this book. Nobody ever says, "I ate healthy for six months, and I feel awful"! It's impossible to eat a proper diet and feel bad about it. This is how we are meant to eat—how we were designed! I have been eating anxiety-free for the past eight years, and while there have been ups and downs, just like in every person's life, I feel so so so good about how I have nourished my body, and I have results to support that.

Life is short; I don't want to miss magical moments. I want to be present in the moment and undistracted by anxiety. I want this for you, too. We can do it together.

Caution: The intent of this book is to provide information of a general nature for educational purposes. It is *not* intended to be used as a substitute for medical care. Never adjust or stop medications without first consulting your doctor. If you are taking medication, always consult your doctor before taking nutritional supplements, in order to prevent adverse reactions.

If you are thinking about suicide, you should seek professional care immediately. You should also seek medical care if you cannot work or maintain relationships, if you feel depressed, or if you find yourself abusing drugs, alcohol, or other substances. You may wish to consider taking medications under the advice and supervision of a medical doctor.

PART I

FOOD AS MEDICINE

CHAPTER 1

Neuroprotective Nutritional Strategies for Reducing Anxiety

Eating to protect your brain is a critical strategy in addressing anxiety and other emotional and mental conditions. You may even feel relief immediately. Science has shown us that if our brain chemistry is right, it will work with equilibrium—meaning, without anxiety. Address the nutritional deficiencies in the body, fix the brain chemistry, and a human body won't suffer with constant anxiety.

WHAT IS ANXIETY?

In 1936, the pioneering endocrinologist Hans Selye defined stress as the "non-specific response of the body to any demand for change."[1] In the decades since then, we have learned a lot more about what happens in our bodies when we feel stressed and recover from stress. Among other things, we know that anxiety is a constant, uncontrollable stress response, where we feel like we are in imminent danger even if no danger is present.

The effects of chronic stress on our health are profound. Researchers have linked ongoing stress to a number of diseases ranging from cardiovascular disease to diabetes, depression, anxiety, and even various cancers. Anxiety is a complex emotional state, a combination of feelings of fear and thoughts of worry. It is often accompanied by instability or tension and associated with an apprehensive anticipation of a future threat.

Anxiety is actually a normal and adaptive natural human emotion, but constant and higher levels of it felt persistently can cause abnormal behaviors and become pathological. Anxiety disorders are among the most common classes of mental disorders.

Physical symptoms of anxiety include having difficulty breathing, elevated blood pressure, heart palpitations, fatigue, sweating, headaches, lightheadedness, digestive problems such as diarrhea and nausea, wobbly "jelly" legs, restlessness, trembling, insomnia, hyperthermia, and dizziness. Mental symptoms include racing thoughts, inability to set aside worry, unwanted thoughts, lack of concentration, hypervigilance, and irritability. Responses to sound, temperature changes, crowds, movement, bright or flickering lights—and other sensory stimuli—may be out of proportion to the impact of the event. This may make us want to run and hide. Mind and body are one and "feed" each other, so thoughts can lead to physical changes and physical changes can lead to anxious thoughts.

Anxiety is involved in many psychiatric disorders, including depression, phobias, panic attacks, obsessive-compulsive disorder, and post-traumatic stress. Furthermore, anxiety disorders often go hand in hand with depressive disorders.[2] For those with anxiety, especially those with an anxiety disorder, there is a worsening in quality of life. Behaviorally, anxiety can lead to substance abuse as individuals attempt to numb themselves to their feelings—everything from overeating to alcohol and drug abuse.

CAUSES OF ANXIETY

There are many causes of anxiety, according to the experts. For the sake of this book's focus on nutritional strategies and recipes to overcome it, I will break them down to physical deficiencies, with the understanding that, of course, there are mental and emotional causes for anxiety too. Nutritional strategies should be used as complements to receiving health care from providers such as physicians and counselors.

Sources of anxiety include:

- *Anxiogenic foods:* Foods that produce anxiety are known as anxiogenic foods. These trigger anxiety straightaway because of how they upset the nervous system. (I will discuss these types of food in Chapter 4.)

  Poor diet is linked to anxiety and depression. Studies have shown that people with mood disorders often have diets that are low in fruits and vegetables and high in fat and sugar.[3]

- *Nutritional deficiency:* The body needs proper levels of certain vitamins and minerals to function in harmony; they are fundamental for our neurotransmitters. If you are anxious, you may also be deficient in magnesium, folate, zinc, amino acids, omega-3 fatty acids, vitamin D, B-complex vitamins, iron, iodine, and selenium.

  A deficiency of a vital nutrient can be caused by a person not eating enough of the right foods or having a digestive system that is unable to function properly. Disordered eating (e.g., overeating, anorexia, bulimia) can also cause malnutrition. I know that when all I ate were fast foods and processed foods, my body was lacking in many essential nutrients. There are significant correlations between anxiety/ depression and food addiction.[4]

A nutritional deficiency can also cause low levels of serotonin, a neurotransmitter that has been considered to be involved in the cause of many disease states, and of gamma-aminobutyric acid (GABA), a neurotransmitter necessary for relaxation, reduction of stress, and sleep. Low levels of GABA may make us feel edgy and irritable.

- *Glycemic imbalance:* Foods that are high on the glycemic index (GI) raise your blood sugar rapidly. Common culprits are white bread, soda, and sugary foods. A "high GI" diet may worsen your mood.[5] If you eat too much refined sugar for too many years, this can cause an imbalance.

- *Obesity:* Obesity is an underlying risk factor for many chronic health conditions and has been associated with increased oxidative stress. Good news: The recipes and foods in this book will help you achieve and maintain a healthy body composition. (Remember, however, that everyone has a different ideal weight at which their body is thriving.) These foods also are a significant source of antioxidant polyphenols and vitamin C, which offer protection against obesity-related health conditions.[6]

- *Lack of sleep/insomnia:* Sleep is like food. It nourishes our bodies and restores them. A lack of sleep is both a contributing factor to, and a symptom of, anxiety.

- *Adrenal "burnout" or fatigue:* When the adrenal glands are spent of their resources and subsequently unable to provide adequate quantities of hormones, primarily cortisol, to respond to our routine needs for them, we experience adrenal fatigue. This condition may be due to chronic stress (which uses up reserves of adrenal hormones) or infections that interfere with production of adrenal hormones. The adrenal glands are located on top of each kidney. If you have adrenal burnout, the recipes in this book will help you recover from it.

- *Sedentary lifestyle:* Being sedentary and prolonged time spent sitting puts us at higher risk for anxiety, according to a meta-analysis of nine studies. One theory is that a sedentary lifestyle causes central nervous system arousal, sleep disturbances, or poor metabolic health, leading to anxiety.[7]

- *Drug and alcohol abuse:* Substance abuse can intensify feelings of sadness, hopelessness, and loneliness, and also puts oxidative stress on the body.

- *Nicotine use:* Nicotine is naturally occurring in plants of the nightshade family, which includes tobacco (*Nicotiana tabacum*). While it has some therapeutic benefits, it's highly addictive and can cause withdrawal when you stop using it. One study found that people with anxiety often self-medicate with nicotine because it eases some symptoms in the short term, but long-term usage "leads to increased baseline severity of anxiety disorder symptoms."[8]

  Common ingredients in cigarettes are another problem: acetone, acetic acid, ammonia, arsenic, benzene, carbon monoxide, formaldehyde, lead, naphthalene, tar, and toluene. The American Lung Association states that there are approximately 600 ingredients in cigarettes, and "when burned, they create more than 7,000 chemicals."[9] These neurotoxins put immediate stress on the nervous system, cause instant oxidative stress, and weaken the immune system.

- *Constant pressure/exposure to psychological stress:* Aside from the biological causes of anxiety, such as nutritional deficiencies, anxiety can also be the result of psychological stress from constant abuse, unresolved childhood trauma, not being loved by your parents, financial hardship, relationship conflicts, sudden loss, and circumstances that are hard to accept.

Prolonged periods of stress, such as you might experience on the job or during a divorce, can deplete your levels of neurotransmitters and cortisol. Having an elevated level of corticotropin-releasing hormone is the main cause of our depressive and anxious symptoms.[10] High, prolonged cortisol releases cause anxiety and fatigue and will interfere with the body's ability to heal.

Our bodies need to be able to release cortisol to survive, because cortisol helps control blood pressure, metabolize glucose (for energy), and reduce inflammation. The key to restoring cortisol levels naturally is to shift your body from its stress response to its relaxation response and to nourish it with the right foods and possibly supplements—which we will explore in the next couple of chapters.

If you believe you have adrenal burnout or cortisol insufficiency, there is a saliva test you can take at home, late at night, when cortisol levels are generally lower. Your health-care provider can recommend a source for this test or provide you with a kit.

- *Oxidative stress (free radical damage):* **Studies reveal that oxidative stress is associated with numerous psychiatric troubles, including pathologically high anxiety.[11]** The production of unstable molecules known as free radicals can be detrimental to our cells, inducing damage to our DNA and RNA. Free radicals contain oxygen that is missing an electron and wants to steal one from other molecules, such as the lipids in cellular membranes. This damage is a key factor in the aging process.

Where does this fit with anxiety? Well, because of its higher oxygen requirement, poor antioxidant defenses, and lipid-rich constitution, the brain is considered particularly susceptible to oxidative stress.[12] Oxidative stress alters overall brain activity, making us more likely to feel anxious, and is a major cause of inflammation.

Long-term oxidative stress comes from foods high in bad fats and refined sugar, especially processed foods; exposure to radiation; excessive alcohol consumption; cigarettes or other tobacco products; some medications; pollution; and exposure to pesticides or industrial chemicals.

- *Inflammation:* Researchers have established links between anxiety and inflammation as well as the reverse. Associations have also been made between reduction of anxiety and anti-inflammatory dietary patterns, such as the high intake of fruits and vegetables.[13]

- *Cognitive decline:* Elderly people may feel anxious when their cognitive function is reduced.[14] Dementia is also associated with alterations of brain chemistry. It's too complex a subject to explore in depth here, but our best chance of maintaining good cognitive function is to take care of our brains when we're young.

- *Poor gut health:* The gut and brain are interconnected. Some neurotransmitters, such as serotonin, are "manufactured" in the intestines, and water-soluble vitamins are synthesized by our symbiotic gut bacteria (aka probiotics). If the gut is not functioning optimally, the body and brain are not properly nourished. An unhappy gut equals an unhappy nervous system and a brain that is not energized.

- *Long periods of fasting:* I was shocked to discover that fasting can cause anxiety in some people. After all, so many people have gotten into intermittent fasting these days, and many experts recommend it. Depriving yourself of food for an extended period of time can raise your levels of cortisol, the main stress hormone.[15] Yet research has found that intermittent fasting does offer some health benefits. Those of us who experience symptoms of anxiety and depression must approach fasting with caution. You can experiment with it to discover how it personally affects you.

- *Other diseases and suffering:* Living with chronic panic, constant headaches and migraines, asthma, irritable bowel syndrome (IBS), cancer, and so on can cause stress and anxiety. But one's mood can also worsen the *outcome* of many of these conditions as well.[16]

- *Antidepressants and antianxiety medication:* This information may be shocking to you. It was to me. Personally, I believe medication can be helpful for some people in some situations. However, many antidepressant and antianxiety drugs have been shown to *worsen* anxiety and depression, as a side effect.[17] Furthermore, all medications have limitations. Common side effects of antidepressant medicines include nausea, increased appetite and weight gain, sexual problems such as erectile dysfunction and decreased orgasm, fatigue and drowsiness, and insomnia, to name only a few. Moreover, some data also indicate that antidepressants may promote suicide.[18] As such, many people are now exploring alternative methods for anxiety prevention and treatment.

NEUROPROTECTIVE FOODS AND THE EFFECT OF FOOD ON ANXIETY

Food can reduce anxiety, and certain foods do *cause* anxiety. If we look at the nutritional composition of any food, we can know if it is anxiolytic (reduces anxiety), neutral, or anxiogenic (causes anxiety).

Consider the common diet shown here. It would likely lead you to develop anxiety and depression, along with other health issues—even though it may seem healthy on the surface because it has a few veggies and protein in it.

- *Breakfast:* A fruit smoothie containing fruit, fruit juice, and water. (A healthy smoothie is great, but if there are no vegetables in it, it's just pure sugar!)

- *Morning snack:* A bagel slathered with margarine. (Bagels have sugar, wheat, and possibly other additives. Margarine is full of trans fats—not ideal.)

- *Lunch:* A bowl of pasta or white rice with vegetables. (The vegetables are good, but white, refined pasta is not as good for you as pasta with more fiber and protein, like beans. White rice is not as good for you as brown rice, which has more fiber.)

- *Afternoon snack:* A granola bar or cookies or gummy candies made with sugar or high-fructose corn syrup.

- *After-school meal:* A bowl of white pasta; it may include meat.

- *Dinner:* A plate of white rice or spaghetti; it may include meat.

- *Evening snack:* Cookies or toast. (By now, blood sugar and insulin levels have spiked and fallen several times today.)

- *Beverages throughout the day:* Two liters of water, a cup of juice, a cup of lactose-free dairy milk, energy drinks, and two cups of coffee.

In the remainder of this chapter, we are going to be looking at nutritional strategies for easing anxiety using food as medicine. I will address how we can take care of our nervous, immune, endocrine, and digestive systems. You will learn about the foods and supplements that have been scientifically evaluated for their anxiety-reducing potential, especially neuroprotective foods.

Neuroprotective foods are so named because they protect our nerve cells against damage. Eating them promotes the body's own natural processes of recovery and regeneration of elements of the nervous system. Among other things, these foods help to nourish the brain so it can do its job of maintaining and regulating the balance in every system of your body.

Neurologists coined the phrase *neuroprotective therapy* to describe treatments for serious ailments of the brain that result from damage to neurons or problems with neurotransmission—either too much or too little excitement. Common neuroprotective treatments are glutamate antagonists—which limit excitation of the neurons—and antioxidants, which help us avoid free radical damage (oxidative stress). Polyphenols, micronutrients that we get through certain plant-based foods, are recognized as offering neuroprotection.[19]

I believe we should fully embrace this concept as a strategy for managing anxiety. Every time we eat, we can ask ourselves, *Am I getting neuroprotection from this food?*

Wow, that question is powerful! It helps us to remember how much is under our control. I love visualizing that my food is either protecting my brain or challenging my brain. It helps me make excellent, self-supporting decisions before every meal.

When we eat in a neuroprotective way, we are supporting the chemical messengers in the brain that transmit signals from cell to cell (the neurotransmitters) and also activate the glands in the endocrine system to release various hormones that regulate our physiological functions. There are more than 40 neurotransmitters in the human nervous system; some of the most important for regulating emotions are serotonin, dopamine, adrenaline, and GABA.

An abnormal level of any neurotransmitter can lead to a mental disorder, including clinical anxiety and depression. If we run out of a given neurotransmitter, the balance of our brain chemistry can be thrown off as the body tries to compensate.

Nutrients are the building blocks the brain and gut use to build neurotransmitters. When we eat, the nutrients we consume have an effect on the levels of our various neurotransmitters; food can trigger a neurotransmitter release. If our neurotransmitters are operating properly, they create a healthy nervous system that has natural checks and balances built into it in the form of inhibitory (calming) and excitatory (stimulating) chemical messengers.

The recipes and foods in this book are designed to help you heal your body and restore your emotional equilibrium. Eating this way will provide you with a diet that is antioxidant-rich and anti-inflammatory. By nourishing your body properly, you will be reducing oxidative stress and fostering a sense of calm. You will also be taking really good care of your brain by providing it with the omega-3 fatty acids and amino acids it needs to function optimally.

Now you will learn the nine key nutritional principles for nourishing your nervous system. The positive thing about this list is that it includes plenty of options. There's no need to attempt to do all of them at once—just doing one of these things can drastically reduce symptoms. So go ahead and just try one; then, if your anxiety level hasn't changed, try another one. Keep going until you have restored emotional equilibrium. You may feel markedly better after following only one or a few of these principles, or all of them!

PRINCIPLE #1. EAT TO PRESERVE GUT HEALTH AND ESTABLISH A HEALTHY MICROBIOME

Good gut health is everything! The brain-gut relationship determines a lot when it comes to anxiety. For good gut health, we need good bacteria living in our systems. The presence and type of microorganisms influence what the gut is able to digest and absorb, and also affect the degree of inflammation throughout the body. This, in turn, contributes to our moods and energy level. The biochemical relationship and signaling that goes on between the cognitive and emotional centers in the brain and the gastrointestinal tract is known as the gut-brain axis.

The importance of the gut-brain connection is also gaining traction among mental health researchers because of multiple studies that show people with anxiety have a different gut microbiome than those who do not![20] Furthermore, according to researchers at RMIT University in Melbourne, Australia, "An influence of gut microbiota on behaviour is becoming increasingly evident, as is the extension to effects on tryptophan and serotonin metabolism. There is regulation of tryptophan and serotonin in the gut by the resident microbiota, and recent studies show that low-to-no gut microbiota increases levels of tryptophan and serotonin and modifies central higher order behaviour."[21]

Microbiome is a term that means "the entire balance of microorganisms in a particular environment." In regard to the gut microbiome, as defined by molecular biologist Joshua Lederberg, it is defined as the totality of microorganisms, including bacteria, viruses, protozoa, and fungi, and their collective genetic material present in the gastrointestinal tract.[22]

This information about anxiety and gut health is so empowering to me; as someone who has suffered anxiety, I didn't know I was at a disadvantage because my microbiome was not right. I had no clue that this meant I would be deficient in some essential nutrients! Among other things gut microbes do is to synthesize vitamins from our food—and make hundreds of neurotransmitters, including 90 to 95 percent of the serotonin the body uses. Serotonin is involved in basic physiological processes like learning, memory, mood, and sleep.[23] As soon as we can replenish this, we can start to feel a whole lot better.

To me, this suggests we ought to help out our guts and feed them the right things to balance the gut microbiome. And it raises an interesting question: Which comes first, an unhealthy gut (due to poor eating and stress) or anxiety (which causes an unhealthy gut)?

An example of gut-brain communication being a two-way street may be irritable bowel syndrome (IBS). There have been cases where IBS causes anxiety and cases where anxiety causes IBS! IBS symptoms can include abdominal pain, bloating, gas, and other digestion issues.

What's interesting is that for many years the medical field did not fully acknowledge the connection between mood and food. But lately, things have changed, and nobody denies it anymore. "Put simply, what you eat directly affects the structure and function of your brain and, ultimately, your mood," says Eva Selhub, M.D., a contributing editor for the *Harvard Health Blog*. "Like an expensive car, your brain functions best when it gets only premium fuel." Meaning our brain functions best when we feed it quality food. She continues, "Unfortunately, just like an expensive car, your brain can be damaged if you ingest anything other than premium fuel. If substances from 'low-premium' fuel (such as what you get from processed or refined foods) get to the brain, it has little ability to get rid of them."[24]

Foods that support helpful microorganisms in the gut are known as prebiotics. (For more information, see Chapter 3.) Eating more complex carbs (whole grains, vegetables, and fruits) and fewer simple carbs (foods containing refined sugar and white flour) can contribute to better gut health. Also, because complex carbohydrates are metabolized more slowly, they help us maintain an even blood sugar level, which gives us a calmer feeling.

You can help replenish the good bacteria in your microbiome through probiotic foods and supplements. You get probiotics naturally when you eat fermented foods like vegetables, cucumbers, pickles, sauerkraut, and kimchi (just make sure they don't have sugar and preservatives added). Kombucha, miso, tempeh, and sourdough contain probiotics. Probiotics are also present in raw milk and raw or fermented milk products, including cheese, kefir, and yogurt. It's important to note, however, that probiotics are destroyed by pasteurization, so be aware when choosing your yogurt and other similar foods.[25]

Personally, I now take probiotic supplements daily to help maintain the quality of my gut microbiome. I feel this helps so much. I feel so much happier and truly more peaceful having a healthy gut. Science seems to be coming in that backs up this strategy. In fact, one systematic review in 2019 examined studies that treated anxiety through regulating the microbiome, either through probiotic use or dietary methods. The researchers found that more than half of the studies "showed that regulating intestinal flora can effectively improve anxiety symptoms." Most impressive to me was that "80 percent of studies that conducted the non-probiotic interventions were effective." They concluded, "In the clinical treatment of anxiety symptoms, in addition to the use of psychiatric drugs for treatment, we can also consider regulating intestinal flora to alleviate anxiety symptoms. Especially for patients with somatic diseases who are not suitable for the application of psychiatric drugs for anxiety treatment, probiotic methods and/or non-probiotic ways . . . can be applied flexibly according to clinical conditions."[26]

PRINCIPLE #2. EAT AND DRINK ONLY NONTOXIC FOODS AND BEVERAGES—AND DO A DETOX, IF NECESSARY

If you know or guess that your body is overloaded with toxins, a detox is a good idea. You would throw out a bucket of dirty water entirely before you began adding clean water to it, wouldn't you?

I suggest doing a full-body detox, which includes a gut cleanse and liver cleanse, so you can lower the toxic burden in the body, give the lymphatic system a chance to restore itself, and let the gut heal so it can absorb nutrients properly. A toxic buildup can lead to anxiety, depression, and fatigue because your gut can't properly absorb the nutrients you are giving it.

When I was sick, I underwent a major detox for three months. This was what I needed to heal my gut and restore balance throughout my body, as well as to dissolve the tumor from my neck. Some people need more or less time. I recommend working with an integrative doctor, nutritionist, or naturopath to do this. Detoxification may not be fun initially, but it is worth it ultimately; it is the best feeling to know that your body is pure. Organs of the elimination system that can benefit from detoxification support include the liver, kidneys, and intestines.

These days, I detox only once a year. For this, I use the Aloe and Colloidal Silver Protocol described in Chapter 3 (see p. 69). You must decide which detox plan is right for you, if any, and if you need to detox, please do a detox. Clean out your "murky water," so you can add in all the good clean stuff and build yourself a nice new body from the inside out.

If you consume something and feel concerned about toxins afterward (for example, high-mercury seafood, fast food, or alcohol), you can consume a clay drink or chlorophyll water. Bentonite clay is ash that has accumulated from volcanoes over millions of years. It binds with heavy metals in the body and helps us to eliminate them from the body. You simply need to drink one teaspoon of bentonite clay mixed in two cups of water. For chlorophyll water, add one serving to a tall glass of water. Both waters are safe enough to incorporate as part of a daily routine.

Starting immediately, you should make a commitment to eat and drink only nontoxic foods and beverages. In Chapter 2, "Top 10 Foods to Reduce Anxiety," you'll find a list of the best foods to focus on eating and why. Start incorporating as many foods from this list into your diet as possible, then observe how eating different foods makes you feel, not just at the moment, but the next hour and the next day. Increasingly, modified diets such as this one are being used to treat behavioral and mood disorders such as anxiety! It's been common across all the research I've done that diets low in sugar and high in fatty acids are recommended.[27]

Just be sure to buy organic and non-GMO ingredients and packaged food. It is important. Fewer pesticides equals less damage done to our DNA and nervous system. The body cannot process pesticides and herbicides well; we take them in, and the body reacts to them as poisons, which often leads to oxidative stress and inflammation. Check out the EWG's Dirty Dozen at www.ewg.org for more information on the produce most likely to contain pesticide residue.

In Chapter 4, "The Most Neurotoxic Foods on the Planet," you'll find an explanation of which foods and types of food products to avoid. Drastically cut back on these—if not altogether eliminating them from your meals—to reduce anxiety. Foods on this list are poisons that have been proven to wreak havoc on the body, causing everything from gut imbalance to nervous system damage and inflammation. These foods add stress to the body, and it's time we let them go.

Let's also not underestimate the importance of purified water. Unfortunately, our water systems these days are contaminated with chlorine, fluoride, and even pharmaceutical drugs that were poured down the drain. I recommend everyone have a water purifier in their home. I have a hydrogen water filter, which helps me maintain gut health. People with anxiety have less hydrogen in their guts, and we need hydrogen for optimum digestion.[28] I have found this to be the most effective water filter I have ever owned. Check it out in the resources section.

PRINCIPLE #3. EAT TO REPLENISH YOUR NEUROTRANSMITTERS

You want to be sure to eat foods that give your brain plentiful reserves of neurotransmitters, chiefly serotonin, dopamine, and gamma-aminobutyric acid (GABA).

- **Serotonin.** Serotonin is known as one of the brain's "happy chemicals." If you have a shortage of serotonin, you may feel sad, depressed, or generally low; have low energy; experience negative thoughts; crave sweets and comfort foods; lose interest in sex; or be tense, irritable, and anxious. As previously mentioned, about 95 percent of the serotonin your body needs to function is produced inside your gastrointestinal tract. The good news is that once your gut is healthy and your microbiome balanced, then all you need to do is eat the right foods and supplements to replenish your serotonin levels.

How to increase it: To be clear, you can't get serotonin directly from food, but you can get tryptophan, an amino acid that's converted to serotonin in your brain. There have been many studies that link the effects of tryptophan to improvements in affective (mood) disorders. A 19-day study of 60 women aged 45 to 65 found that 1 gram of tryptophan per day led to increased energy and improved happiness.[29]

Foods that contain an abundance of the amino acid tryptophan are chicken, turkey, eggs, organic dairy (such as cheese and milk), fish, peanuts, pumpkin seeds, sesame seeds, spinach, parsley, watercress, cremini mushrooms, beet greens, bamboo shoots, and asparagus.

- **Dopamine.** Dopamine is another of the brain's feel-good neurotransmitters. As part of the brain's reward system, it's released when we do things like eat food that we crave or have sex. It is also associated with our sleep-wake cycles. This important neurochemical boosts mood, motivation, and focus and helps regulate our emotional responses.

   People with low levels of dopamine may be more prone to addiction. A person seeking pleasure via food, drugs, or alcohol needs higher and higher levels of dopamine to take the same pleasure in the reward.[30] It's a vicious cycle, one that I know very well because, for a time, I was addicted to sugary foods and fast foods.

   If you suspect that you are suffering from dopamine deficiency, consult your doctor. Dopamine levels are easily checked with a simple blood or urine test. A person's mental health, including anxiety and concentration, can be affected even by slightly low levels of dopamine! If you have an addiction to anything, you could have a deficiency in dopamine that you're unaware of.

How to increase it: There are ways to increase your dopamine levels naturally with food, supplements, and self-care activities. You can supplement with tyrosine, an amino acid that converts to dopamine in the body. Foods rich in tyrosine include seeds, nuts, beans, lentils, organic dairy (e.g., milk and cottage cheese), grass-fed meats, fish (e.g., salmon, orange roughy), egg whites, turkey, chicken, shrimp, and non-GMO soy.

A restless night can reduce your dopamine reserves drastically, so proper sleep hygiene is important for reducing anxiety. Remember that sleep, as well as exercise, fuels dopamine production. Stress, on the other hand, drains the brain of dopamine, so do what you can to reduce stress.

Fruits of the *Musa* genus (e.g., bananas and plantains) and the *Persea americana* species (avocado) contain high levels of both tyrosine and tryptophan, so they are good for replenishing dopamine *and* serotonin.[31]

- **GABA.** Anxiety signifies a dysregulation of the nervous system. Normally, GABA counterbalances the actions of the excitatory neurotransmitter glutamate. They are paired; one ramps us up, and the other calms us down. Without GABA, we are in go mode. So when we drink a caffeinated beverage like coffee, which gives us a jolt of energy, the release of GABA is being inhibited in the brain. A deficiency of GABA can lead to anxiety, stress, insomnia, trouble concentrating, forgetfulness, and depression; it's even been linked to substance abuse.[32]

  How to increase it: GABA is considered a *dietary neurotransmitter* because, although it is made in the

brain, it is also present in some of the beverages
we consume, like tea (especially green tea), and
in some of the foods we eat, such as beans (fava,
soy, lentil, and others), walnuts, citrus fruits, fish
(halibut, shrimp), broccoli, potatoes, tomatoes, and
berries. Also, try fermented foods, which are rich
in probiotics, like kimchi, sauerkraut, and kefir.
Many traditional foods produced by microbial
fermentation contain GABA. The main precursor
nutrient of GABA is glucose, which is plentiful in
healthy carbohydrates. You should also know about
theanine and arginine, two amino acids that boost
the action of GABA.

GABA supplements are available, but there
are other ways to increase your levels. Consider
supplementation with vitamin B_6, a cofactor in the
synthesis of GABA, and with probiotic bacteria.
Lactobacillus strains, such as *L. rhamnosus*, *L.
paracasei*, and *L. brevis*, and *Lactococcus lactis*, are said
to be ideal.[33]

Caution: If you are taking prescription medication,
GABA supplements may be contraindicated. Check
with your doctor first.

Principle #4. Eat to Overcome Nutritional Deficiencies

Nutritional deficiencies can mean your brain does not have the
building blocks it needs to function optimally. You need amino
acids, which come from protein, to build a healthy body. Also,
several of the B-complex vitamins, including thiamin, riboflavin,
niacin, vitamin B_6, folate, and vitamin B_{12}, are needed as cofactors
for the synthesis of neurotransmitters in the gut.

Iron deficiency can cause anxiety because it reduces the
oxygen available to body tissues.[34] Lack of iron strongly affects
the balance between excitatory and calming brain chemicals,
such as glutamate (excitatory) and GABA (calming)—for which

reason eating iron-rich foods is imperative for treating anxiety. Your doctor can test to see if you are iron deficient.

Most of these can be taken in from whole foods we eat. That said, taking supplements is also a powerful way to put the nutrients that reduce anxiety straight into your body with little effort on your part. Especially when your anxiety is related to chronic stress or malnourishment, it's reasonable to consider enacting this strategy. See Chapter 3, "Top Antianxiety Supplements," for a list of ideas about which supplements to try.

To function adequately, the central nervous system requires a number of amino acids found in protein, and a deficiency of these has a link to stress and anxiety and depression.[35] One way to improve your neurotransmitters overall, therefore, is simply to boost your protein intake! When you eat protein, it's broken down into amino acids, which are then used to help your body with various processes such as regulating immune function, nourishing the brain, building muscle, and assisting with mood, intestinal function, and fertility. However, be aware that too much protein can result in elevated levels of amino acids and their by-products (for example, ammonia, homocysteine, and asymmetric dimethylarginine), which may be pathogenic factors for neurological disorders, oxidative stress, and cardiovascular disease. An optimal balance among amino acids in the diet and circulation is crucial for whole-body homeostasis.[36]

Your body needs nine essential amino acids—histidine, isoleucine, leucine, lysine, methionine, phenylalanine, threonine, tryptophan, and valine—to function properly.[37] (See the section "Amino Acids" in Chapter 3 for more information.) These foods are the most common sources of essential amino acids:

- *Lysine:* grass-fed meat, eggs, non-GMO soy, black beans, quinoa, and pumpkin seeds
- *Histidine:* meat, fish, poultry, nuts, seeds, and whole grains
- *Threonine:* cottage cheese, wheat germ, non-GMO soy, beans, nuts, and grains

PRINCIPLE #5. EAT MORE MAGNESIUM-RICH FOODS

One of the causes of anxiety is being deficient in magnesium. You could get a blood test if you aren't sure of your own levels. The anxiolytic potential of magnesium has been demonstrated in studies.

Magnesium modulates activity in the hypothalamic-pituitary-adrenal axis, which is a central communication highway for the stress response system. The brain region of the hypothalamus tells the pituitary gland that it's time for you to feel stressed, and the pituitary switches on the adrenal glands, which release cortisol. That's great if you're running from a deranged madman carrying a rifle and threatening to shoot you, but it's not great if you're at a party with a group of friends or getting ready to go to work on Monday morning. Activation of this adrenal axis instigates adaptive autonomic, neuroendocrine, and behavioral responses to cope with the demands of a stressor, and it also increases anxiety.[38]

Interestingly, it's been shown that people who are sleep deprived are likely to be deficient in magnesium.[39] We know that increasing magnesium intake through foods can up your dopamine levels, making you feel more relaxed and satisfied. You can find it in foods such as beans, seeds, nuts, soybeans (edamame, tofu, and so on), whole grains, wild rice, cacao, chickpeas, lentils, salmon, bananas, avocados, and spinach.

Consuming magnesium-rich food or taking magnesium supplements has been demonstrated to reduce the expression of anxiety-related behavior and put more control in our hands.[40] Isn't this information utterly relieving?

PRINCIPLE #6. EAT MORE OMEGA-3 FATS

One of the most common causes of anxiety is being deficient in omega-3 fatty acids. You can get a blood test done to check your levels if you aren't sure. This is something my own blood work revealed I was deficient in, and I immediately felt better once I started to eat more salmon and take fish oil capsules.

Omega-3 fatty acids include docosahexaenoic acid (DHA), alpha-lipoic acid (ALA), and eicosapentaenoic acid (EPA). DHA is an omega-3 fatty acid that is a primary structural component of the human brain, cerebral cortex, skin, and retina, and its deficiency is linked to several neurocognitive disorders and behaviors linked to anxiety and depression.[41] Notably, low levels of DHA are associated with generalized anxiety,[42] whereas supplementation with DHA has been shown to have anxiolytic effects.[43]

Primary sources of DHA are fish, including anchovies, salmon, herring, mackerel, tuna, trout, mussels, oysters, Atlantic cod, caviar, snow crab, tiger prawn, barramundi, clams, and halibut; grass-fed red meat; and turkey. Eggs naturally contain small amounts of DHA. If you're vegan or just interested in getting your omega-3s from plant-based sources, you can get DHA from spirulina, a type of blue-green algae. I add spirulina to my Genius Smoothie every day, and I'm not even vegan. You could also take a fish oil supplement. I do both.

Because vegetarians and vegans do not eat fish, they consume virtually no EPA and DHA. However, vegetarians and vegans often eat a diet rich in the plant-derived omega-3 fatty acid alpha-linolenic acid (ALA). In one study, researchers at the University of California, Los Angeles, were trying to better understand how turmeric and its active component, curcumin, support brain health. They found that consuming curcumin actually increases the cellular machinery necessary to convert ALA into EPA and DHA.[44] This is why turmeric (and its active compound, curcumin) can be another vegan source for DHA.

Other plant-based sources of DHA are certain algae, seaweed, chia seeds, hempseeds, flaxseeds, walnuts, strawberry, broccoli, edamame, kidney beans, pumpkin seeds, soybeans, avocado, coconut and coconut oil, sunflower seeds and sunflower oil, and olive oil and olives.

PRINCIPLE #7. EAT MORE ANTIOXIDANTS

Researchers at the State University of New York at Buffalo found that anxiety is associated with a low antioxidant state in the body. Furthermore, antioxidants elevate mood immediately and provide long-lasting health![45] Antioxidants are compounds in food that inhibit oxidation. People with anxiety and constant stress have an increased amount of oxidation in the body, and eating antioxidants reverses this process. Oxidation is caused by many factors, including chronic stress and anxiety. Oxidative imbalance in the body leads to anxiety.[46]

Oxidation is a chemical reaction that produces free radicals, leading to chain reactions that damage the cells. But antioxidants are like superhero molecules that come in and stand up to the free radicals that are villainizing the body. Antioxidants are found in fruits and vegetables and are segregated into these three groups: vitamins, phenolic compounds, and carotenoids. For example, vitamins A, C, and E are all antioxidants. Hydroxytyrosol, which is a phenolic compound drawn from the olive tree and found in olive oil, is said to be the most powerful natural antioxidant currently known.

You consume the antioxidants you need every time you eat plant-based foods: fruits, vegetables, nuts, and seeds. Some are higher in antioxidants than others. Fortunately for you, the recipes in this book are *all* high in antioxidants. Everything in the top 10 list of foods to reduce anxiety in this book offers a generous supply of antioxidants.

A group of researchers from the department of nutrition at the University of Oslo's Institute of Basic Medical Sciences in Norway did an incredible study in 2010 of more than 3,000 foods to find out which were the highest in antioxidants. These foods constitute the Antioxidant Food Table.[47] This database is, to the best of my knowledge, the most comprehensive database of antioxidant foods ever published. It shows without a doubt that plant-based foods introduce significantly more antioxidants into our diet than non-plant foods.

There are several-thousand-fold differences in the antioxidant content of different foods. Spices and herbs are some of the most antioxidant-rich ingredients, and some levels are exceptionally high. Clove, mint, cinnamon, oregano, thyme, and rosemary are the highest! Nuts and seeds were the next most antioxidant-rich, with the level in walnuts being off the chart, followed by the level in pecans, and then in sunflower seeds and chestnuts. Berries, fruits, vegetables, chocolate, and even coffee were also loaded. I was the most surprised to see that walnuts were the highest of all 3,000 commonly known antioxidant-rich foods!

We know from countless proven studies that a plant-based diet protects against chronic oxidative-stress-related diseases. Nutritive plants contain diverse chemicals and amounts of antioxidants that contribute to incredibly beneficial health effects. The berries, fruits, and vegetables highest in antioxidants according to the table are as follows—and it's a mixture of common ones and some that are quite obscure depending on which continent you reside on:

Top Antioxidant-Rich Foods
(according to the Antioxidant Food Table)

1. Amla (Indian gooseberry), dried

2. Dog rose/rose hips

3. Bilberries

4. African baobab tree, leaves and fruit

5. Zereshk (red sour berries also known as barberries)

6. Moringa

7. Okra/gumbo from Mali (dry flour)

8. Apples, dried

9. Artichokes (tied with blueberries)

10. Blueberries

11. Plums

12. Apricots

13. Kale

14. Chili (tied with prunes)

15. Prunes

16. Strawberries

17. Pomegranates

18. Black olives (tied with dates and mangoes)

19. Dates

20. Mangoes

21. Oranges

22. Papayas

23. Broccoli

Plant-Based Eating vs. Meat-Inclusive Eating

This is always a big debate with any disease: What is better, eating meat or going vegan? There are more antioxidants in plant-based foods, but there are more proteins and omega-3 fatty acids in animal-based foods and seafood. Meat and fish do contain omega-3 fatty acids; however, we *can* get them from plant sources, like chia seeds and flaxseeds. I believe what you eat is your personal choice, and I encourage you to do what is right for you.

Vegans with anxiety should be vigilant to make sure to get sufficient omega-3 fatty acids, and you would want to consider taking B-complex vitamins, especially B_{12}—the reasons are explained in Chapter 3, "Top Antianxiety Supplements." A meat-eater can get all of these nutrients from meat and fish. Even so, I would recommend that meat-eaters make sure to eat a majority plant-based diet, filled with plenty of vegetables, nuts, seeds, and fruits, because of how a plant-based diet protects against chronic oxidative-stress-related anxiety. Plants are generally higher in antioxidant content than meats.

In a study of different foods that were scored for their antidepressant content per serving of 100 grams, vegetables scored the highest (48 percent), followed by organ meats (25 percent), fruits (20 percent), seafood (16 percent), legumes (8 percent), meats (8 percent), nuts and seeds (5 percent), grains (5 percent), and dairy from cows (3 percent).[48] This shows us that we should indeed increase vegetable consumption to experience a natural antidepressant. As we've discussed, anxiety often goes hand in hand with depression.

Personally, I do eat a modest amount of animal protein. I tried to go vegan when I was sick, thinking that was the "right" thing to do, but it made me feel weak, so I reintroduced some animal protein here and there in my meals, and it gave me the strength to heal. A vegan may not understand that, but something similar has happened to a lot of people who have healed brain issues and cancer. Science will show us there are certain nutrients and proteins we get from animal protein that are incredibly beneficial for our health. I certainly do not mean to advocate the consumption of massive portions of meat, just eating the right amount for your body.

PRINCIPLE #8. EAT MORE PLANT-BASED FOODS— RAW FRUITS AND VEGETABLES, ESPECIALLY

We cannot go wrong with a higher plant-based intake that includes vegetables, fruits, nuts, seeds, herbs, and spices. Studies have shown that consuming more plant-based ingredients reduces anxiety and depression because they contain a wide variety of micronutrients critical to physical and mental function, as well as complex carbs and fiber. Plants also help us to stay well hydrated.

There is evidence that people who eat more fruits and vegetables have better mental health, including lower rates of depression, perceived stress, and negative mood.[49] But when surveyed, they also will say that they experience better moods and greater life satisfaction, and have a stronger sense of purpose and fulfillment. If that's not a recommendation for eating more fruits and vegetables, then I don't know what is.

With that said, I don't think it's wise for many of those with depression and anxiety to completely cut out animal foods. Certain nutrients, such as long-chain omega-3 fats, vitamin B_{12}, and heme iron, are found only in animal-based foods such as seafood, meat, eggs, and dairy. As health recommendations have trended toward more plant-based diets, one must consider the higher rates of vitamin B deficiencies in both vegetarian and vegan populations. A recent large study found higher levels of depressive symptoms in vegetarian men.[50]

Furthermore, DHA deficiency is implicated in many neurological disorders, and fish is a primary source of DHA. Vegetarians and vegans have reduced plasma DHA compared to omnivores.[51] You can be a healthy vegan, but I believe it takes more diligence, and you must be vigilant. One study suggested that curcumin (a primary component of turmeric) enhances DHA synthesis, which would be incredibly helpful for those with low DHA due to eating a plant-based diet or who do not consume fish.[52] Personally, I believe that the most balanced way of eating is a plant-rich diet with some modest quantities of meat, eggs, dairy, and seafood.

Aside from eating more plant-based foods in general, you can also benefit from increasing your consumption of raw ones. We know that both cooked fruits and vegetables and raw fresh fruits and vegetables provide the body with nutrients and healing. Raw foods, for the most part, provide us with more nutrients than cooked foods, although some nutrients in foods become more bioavailable when lightly cooked. However, there is evidence to support the mental health benefits of raw fruits and vegetables.

In a 2018 study published in *Frontiers in Medicine*, 422 adults aged 18 to 25 completed an online survey that assessed their typical consumption of raw, cooked, canned, and processed fruits and vegetables and compared it with their mental health, including depressive symptoms, anxiety, negative mood, positive mood, life satisfaction, and flourishing. This study showed that depressive and anxiety symptoms reduced significantly, negative mood decreased, and positive mood and life satisfaction significantly increased when participants ate more raw foods. (However, a flaw in the study is that the researchers did not differentiate between cooked fresh ingredients and canned foods.)

Among the raw foods identified by the study that relate to better mental health, these are the top 10:[53]

1. Carrots

2. Bananas

3. Apples

4. Dark leafy greens, like spinach and kale

5. Grapefruit

6. Lettuce

7. Citrus fruits, like oranges and lemons

8. Berries

9. Cucumbers

10. Kiwifruit

The study concluded: "The cooking and processing of raw foods have the potential to diminish nutrient levels, which likely limits the delivery of nutrients that are essential for optimal emotional functioning." They went on to suggest that increasing raw fruit and vegetable consumption may "provide an accessible adjuvant approach to improving mental health."[54]

Raw fruits, vegetables, nuts, and seeds make excellent snacks and are the ultimate "fast food." Fresh berries make a great dessert. A carrot is so lovely to crunch on, as are apples. They're nature's candy. I encourage us all to snack on more raw foods like this in their wholesome, natural state.

Principle #9. Eat to Reduce Inflammation

Oxidation damages the body. Inflammation is the body's response to repair the damage—and it can get out of control. It's been shown that inflammation in the body causes anxiety but also that anxiety causes inflammation.[55]

You will effortlessly reduce inflammation in your body when you eat foods high in antioxidants, magnesium, omega-3 fatty acids, and amino acids while avoiding toxic foods filled with processed sugar, preservatives, and unnatural additives. The recipes in this book are all anti-inflammatory. If it comes from nature, an ingredient does not usually cause inflammation.

A powerful way to reduce inflammation in your body almost immediately is to eat turmeric (such as in a curry dish) or take a supplement of curcumin, which is a compound in turmeric. Turmeric has been perhaps the most studied spice of all time because of its therapeutic effects as an anti-inflammatory agent against neurodegenerative, cardiovascular, pulmonary, metabolic, autoimmune, and neoplastic diseases.[56]

Turmeric has neuroprotective effects because it's able to reduce inflammatory markers, like cytokines, which have been known to cause anxiety. It also increases blood antioxidant levels, which tend to be low in individuals with anxiety.

Having quick and easy health hacks, such as sprinkling turmeric on your breakfast eggs or taking a daily supplement, can dramatically reduce inflammation in your body.[57]

OTHER WAYS TO REDUCE STRESS AND SOOTHE ANXIETY

We feel anxious when our fight-or-flight stress response is triggered. The activation of the sympathetic nervous system is intended by nature to be followed by the relaxation response, which we can induce by activating the parasympathetic nervous system. If we're anxious, we are more likely to make poor decisions about what we eat. If we're relaxed, hopefully we will make better decisions about what we eat. The following activities, along with an anxiety-free eating plan, can help us relax and recover when we're feeling stressed:

- Spending time in nature
- Prayer
- Meditation

- Talking to a friend
- Exercise—at least 30 minutes per day of moderate activity
- Gratitude—make a list of what you're thankful for before bed or upon waking in the morning
- Aromatherapy with essential oils
- Creating a vision board with goals you set for yourself
- Revisiting your happy memories
- Listening to music
- Sleeping
- Yoga or stretching
- Spiritual healing
- Acupuncture
- Massage
- Acupressure: Pressing on the yin tang pressure point located at the midpoint between your eyebrows can help relieve stress and anxiety. To do this, sit back in a comfortable position. Place your right thumb or forefinger between your eyebrows and hold it there for a few minutes while breathing. Close your eyes and do your best to let go of stress and worry.

* * *

Are you ready to read about the top foods to reduce anxiety? Turn the page, and let's dive right into the science behind these life-changing foods.

CHAPTER 2

The Top 10 Foods to Reduce Anxiety

It's impossible to ignore the science revealing the correlations between what we eat and our mental health. Food has a crucial impact on the brain, nervous system, and endocrine system. In this chapter, we will look at some of the best, most desirable natural ingredients, foods that can help us balance our body chemistry so that we improve our moods, sleep better, reduce our stress, and prevent or soothe anxiety.

In the previous chapter, we looked at several causes for anxiety related to nutrition. Countless studies, for example, have shown that anxiety may be caused by deficiency of magnesium and omega-3 fatty acids, and oxidative stress from free radicals. There are nutritional solutions to all these problems. Based on these studies, I believe that the three most important elements in foods to help reduce anxiety are magnesium, omega-3 fatty acids, and antioxidants.

The items in the top 10 list of foods in this chapter usually contain more than one of these three main types of antianxiety nutrients. For example, the food taking first place, dark leafy greens, is high in both magnesium and antioxidants.

Exciting Development in Nutritional Management of Anxiety

Now more than ever, macronutrients (fats, carbs, and proteins) and micronutrients (minerals, vitamins, and phytochemicals) are topics of interest in neuropsychiatry, the branch of medicine that deals with mental disorders attributable to diseases of the nervous system.[1] The search for foods that balance brain chemistry and replenish neurotransmitters has produced the new interdisciplinary approach of nutritional neuroscience. According to a report in the journal *Nutrients*: "From now on, psychobiotics, different animal foods, fruits, edible plants, roots, and botanicals, will be seen as natural sources of neurotransmitters."[2]

While many people find success with medications that manage their anxiety, I believe that using medication alone without addressing possible nutritional deficiencies is unlikely to lead to the long-term management of symptoms. If someone is taking medication while continuing to eat a poor diet, the underlying physical imbalances just get worse.

The basis of the recipes in this book is organic, natural foods that help you feel your best; I hope to empower you to build your own diet plan from them. The decision of what to eat depends on your bioindividuality—not everyone's body responds the same way to walnuts, or salmon, or cacao, for example. Does your body respond better to omegas from fish or from walnuts? Or a combination of both? For some people, mushrooms are a superfood; other people's bodies react to them like a poison. Balanced eating and respecting your bioindividuality is about finding the nutrition-rich foods that work for you specifically.

Please note that this top 10 list includes foods that are readily available to most people, rather than rarer foods indigenous to remote regions that would be excellent for managing anxiety too.

Before the scientific method existed, knowledge about the therapeutic use of food was passed down through generations by word of mouth. For example, ginger was known to help manage colds and nausea. Although people didn't know the chemical reasons why, they knew it worked. Now that researchers are studying these foods, we know exactly why they have the effects on us that they do. I am sure you will be just as fascinated as I am with the research on their ability to reduce anxiety.

Keep in mind that I recommend taking a bioindividual approach in acting upon this list. Don't just blindly follow the recommendations. Start by paying attention to how eating each of these foods makes you feel—not just in the moment, but in an hour and over the next day. Eat more of the ones that make you feel best.

Are you ready to eat your way to calm? Then read on.

The Top 10 Foods for Reducing Anxiety

1. Dark leafy greens, such as kale, spinach, and parsley

2. Walnuts

3. Turmeric

4. Wild salmon and other fatty fish

5. Avocado

6. Olive oil

7. Coconut oil

8. Broccoli and broccoli sprouts

9. Cacao

10. Ginger

#1 DARK LEAFY GREENS

Dark leafy greens take first place in managing, alleviating, and even preventing anxiety!

Dark leafy greens include:

- Kale
- Spinach
- Parsley
- Lettuce
- Broccoli
- Broccoli sprouts
- Collard greens
- Chard
- Arugula
- Bok choy
- Mustard greens
- Dandelion greens

One of the main reasons dark leafy greens are #1 on the list is that they contain the compound chlorophyll—the pigment that makes plants green—which enhances our tolerance for oxidative stress. One particular study on the antioxidative capacity of chlorophyll isolated from spinach described how it increased the life span of microorganisms by more than 20 percent. The researchers report that "dietary chlorophyll derivatives support the recommendation of nutritionists to eat green vegetables and salads containing high contents of chlorophyll, as this could help to improve human health and prevent diseases."[3]

Another reason dark leafy greens take first place is their high antioxidant level. The level of nutrients in green leafy vegetables with positive bioactive properties is off the charts, which is why countless studies show that symptoms of depression and anxiety can be reduced significantly, and positive mood and life satisfaction increased significantly, when we eat more dark leafy greens.[4]

Dark leafy greens help to protect the brain and support its optimal functioning, preventing cognitive decline. The primary nutrients (including bioactive ones) in dark leafy greens, as well as in green vegetables, include vitamin K (phylloquinone), vitamin C, vitamin E (alpha-tocopherol), beta-carotene, lutein, nitrate, folate, and kaempferol.

Dark leafy greens are also among the best sources of magnesium on earth. Dietary intake of magnesium has been shown to be insufficient in a staggeringly high percentage of Western populations, including 68 percent of American adults[5] and 72 percent of middle-aged French adults.[6] The relationship between magnesium and depression and anxiety states has been well established in studies of the depletion and supplementation of magnesium in animals and humans.[7]

One study included volunteers from more than 40 retirement communities, senior public housing units, and churches and senior centers in the Chicago area. The researchers came to the conclusion that consumption of approximately one serving per day of green leafy vegetables—and other foods rich in phylloquinone (vitamin K_1), lutein, nitrate, folate, alpha-tocopherol (vitamin E), and kaempferol—may help to slow cognitive decline with aging. They noted that "the addition of a daily serving of green leafy vegetables to one's diet may be a simple way to contribute to brain health."[8]

Research shows that increasing our intake of vegetables of every kind can protect against cognitive decline.[9] Dark-green leafy plants, however, give us the strongest protection. A study of aging women found that those consuming the most green leafy vegetables experienced slower decline than women consuming the least amount.[10] A healthy brain almost certainly is going to be less inclined toward mood disorders. I believe that dark leafy greens are a major contributor to my well-being today.

Ways of Incorporating Dark Leafy Greens in Your Anxiety-Free Kitchen

- Use kale, spinach, lettuce, and collard greens as a base for your salads! A combination of all of them makes for one vibrantly green salad bowl.

- Eat them raw.

- Cook them with stir-fried vegetables.

- Add chopped dark leafy greens—especially parsley and spinach—to soups.

- Include them in smoothies and juices.

- Use liquid chlorophyll in your water, juices, smoothies, tea, and/or coffee.

Anxiety-Free Recipes with Dark Leafy Greens

- Superfood Kale Salad

- Master Smoothie

- Super Greens Juice

- Thai Sauteed Greens

#2 WALNUTS

Walnuts are incredibly high in antioxidants. In a Norwegian analysis of thousands of foods, resulting in the Antioxidant Food Table, walnuts tested as having the highest antioxidant content of all nuts, legumes, and grains.[11] Walnuts also contain neuroprotective compounds, including vitamin E, folate, melatonin, several polyphenols, magnesium, and copper. (You can read more about the benefits of copper in Chapter 3.)

Walnuts are a phenomenal source of the good fats that our brains and nervous systems need to reduce anxiety. In fact, walnuts are the *only* tree nut that is an excellent source of ALA, the plant-based omega-3 fatty acid that is essential for our healthy existence. They are one of the best plant food sources of omega-3s around. These good fats help reduce inflammation. One study showed that supplementation with walnuts was able to improve mood in young adults.[12] Another study showed that people who consume walnuts have lower depression scores.[13]

Walnuts have been proven time and time again to have beneficial effects on cognition and overall brain health. Oxidative stress and neuroinflammation play important roles in disorders associated with the brain, like anxiety. Reports suggest there are benefits of a walnut-enriched diet for treating brain disorders and other chronic diseases, due to the compounds in walnuts that protect against oxidative stress and inflammation.[14]

Fun fact: A walnut looks similar to the human brain. The walnut shape represents the left and right hemispheres. The creases on the nut are similar to those of the neocortex. It is no wonder walnuts are known as "brain food."

Ways of Incorporating Walnuts in Your Anxiety-Free Kitchen

- Eat raw walnuts as a snack. The recommended serving size is a small handful.

- Add walnuts to your smoothie.

- Add walnuts to your breakfast oatmeal or chia seed cereal.

- Use walnut oil as a base for salad dressings.

- Sprinkle them on salads.

- Add them to a vegetable stir-fry.

- Eat them with homemade chocolate.

- Make a raw walnut flour by processing whole walnuts in a blender and crust your meat with it.

Anxiety-Free Recipes with Walnuts

- Walnut Butter
- Walnut "Meatballs" with Zoodles
- Walnut-Crusted Chicken Salad
- Smart Cookies

#3 TURMERIC

Turmeric is rich in antioxidants and renowned for being powerfully anti-inflammatory. One of the main reasons turmeric is so highly prized is because it contains the compound curcumin, which is not only anticancer and antidiabetic but also good for the brain. Curcumin helps boost the conversion of the plant-based omega-3 fatty acid ALA into DHA, which is essential to brain function.

Why should we care? Well, dietary deficiency of DHA is linked to the neuropathology of several cognitive disorders, one of which is anxiety. DHA is primarily obtained through diet; however, the efficiency of the conversion of its plant-based dietary precursors is low (which is why we are often advised to take fish oil supplements). A study was performed to determine the molecular mechanisms involved with curcumin and DHA, and it was discovered that it elevates levels of enzymes in both liver and brain tissue.[15]

An overview of studies on curcumin published in the *Indian Journal of Pharmaceutical Sciences* found the following: Curcumin demonstrates neuroprotective action in individuals who have Alzheimer's disease, tardive dyskinesia, major depression, and other related degenerative neurological and psychiatric disorders. In addition to its anti-inflammatory and antioxidant properties, it is a potent inhibitor of reactive astrocyte expression and, thus, prevents cell death. Curcumin also modulates various neurotransmitter levels in the brain.[16]

There have been many great studies on the use of curcumin for treatment of anxiety and other central nervous system disorders.

One stood out to me most. In it, researchers measured anxiety-related behavioral responses and serotonin levels in rodents after prolonged exposure to stress. The subjects received curcumin in doses of 20 milligrams, 50 milligrams, or 100 milligrams once per day for 14 days. Curcumin administration considerably reduced the protective "freezing" response associated with fear and aided the subjects' neurochemical recovery. Overall, the study concluded that curcumin has anxiolytic effects on biochemical and behavioral symptoms associated with anxiety. These researchers even say that "curcumin may be an alternative treatment for preventing anxiety-like behavior associated with PTSD."[17]

Based on a vast amount of evidence, we know that curcumin acts on the brain in multiple ways. I think it is only a matter of time before curcumin is viewed as a legitimate mainstream therapy for various neurological disorders. Wow, food is powerful!

And aren't we fortunate that we don't need a doctor to prescribe turmeric? Just make some curried veggies in your kitchen at home, and you'll be good to go.

Ways of Incorporating Turmeric in Your Anxiety-Free Kitchen

- Add turmeric to everything! Just think *What can I add turmeric to?* before your meal. Add a small sprinkle of turmeric to tea or coffee, to vegetable stir-fry, meat, chicken, fish, scrambled eggs, omelets, soups, and rice and quinoa. It goes so well with both vegetables and meat!

- At home, I use a vegan ghee from Nutiva that has turmeric in it to make Broccoli Popcorn (see p. 190) and stir-fried vegetables.

- If you don't enjoy cooking with turmeric, perhaps because you don't like the flavor or because you worry that it may stain your teeth and hands, you might consider taking a turmeric or curcumin supplement instead of cooking with it.

Anxiety-Free Recipes with Turmeric

- Turmeric Cauliflower Rice
- Walnut-Crusted Chicken
- Vitamin C Blast
- Grounding Lentil Soup with Avocado and Ginger

#4 Wild Salmon (and Other Fatty Fish)

Salmon is in our fourth spot because of the abundance of omega-3s it provides (like other fatty fish). Salmon also contains astaxanthin, a carotenoid antioxidant found to benefit the brain and nervous system. In addition, salmon is high in magnesium, making it an antianxiety trifecta for providing all three of the main nutrients that are proven to help reduce anxiety.

Salmon has anxiolytic-like effects because it is full of long-chain polyunsaturated fatty acids (PUFAs), peptides, polysaccharides, vitamins, minerals, antioxidants, and enzymes. PUFAs, especially, have proven to be helpful for the treatment of mood disorders.[18]

An interesting research study was conducted in which 95 people who were assigned to eat salmon three times a week from September through February were compared with a control group who ate an alternative meal, such as chicken, pork, or beef three times a week. The anxiety of the subjects was assessed at the beginning and end of the study. The salmon-eating group showed significant improvements. These findings suggest that regular salmon consumption can play a positive role in the regulation of emotions in people experiencing anxiety.[19]

You may have noticed that I insist upon wild-caught salmon. Why wild versus farmed? I talk about this more in Chapter 4, as farmed fish is unfortunately one of the worst foods we can eat.

Other fish with fabulous fats that can nourish our brains and reduce anxiety are (given that they are all wild and, in some cases, organically farmed is an exception) tuna, trout, sardines, mackerel, herring, mussels, anchovies, and swordfish.

Ways of Incorporating Wild Salmon in Your Anxiety-Free Kitchen

- Always keep frozen wild salmon in your freezer so you have it ready to go any night of the week.

- Commit to eating wild salmon at least two to three times a week.

- Bake it or fry it in some avocado oil. It's delicious with a little garlic salt and a squeeze of lemon.

- Serve salmon on a dark leafy green salad, or if you are in a pinch for time, a huge bed of broccoli sprouts.

- If you don't like the taste or smell of fish, you may want to consider taking a fish oil supplement.

Anxiety-Free Recipes with Salmon

- Baked Walnut-Crusted Salmon
- Baked Fish with Roasted Vegetables and a Side of Yucca

#5 AVOCADO

Botanically, avocado fruit is a berry with a single large seed. I know you will never look at an avocado the same way again now that you know this, right?

Avocado is known as a superfood because of its exceptional nutritional and phytochemical composition; it is a rich source of potassium, vitamins E and C, and beta-carotene (provitamin A). Moreover, avocados contain a number of minerals, including phosphorus, magnesium, calcium, sodium, iron, and zinc.

Avocado is said to have a neuroprotective effect due to its unique antioxidants, which preferentially impede the generation of free radicals.[20]

Compared to other vegetable oils, avocado oil is high in monounsaturated fatty acids (MUFAs), healthy fats like oleic and palmitoleic acids, and low in PUFAs, like linoleic acid and linolenic acid. Avocado oil proved to increase production of collagen, a protein that is a major component of connective tissue, and decrease inflammation in a study.[21] There aren't many organic avocado oils in the marketplace; I recommend the ones that Nutiva distributes.

In terms of its total fat composition, avocado oil is most similar to olive oil. Oleic acid is the principal fatty acid in avocado, comprising 45 percent of its total content.[22]

Avocados are notable for being potassium-rich. A single serving provides 60 percent more potassium than an equal amount of banana.[23] Potassium can reduce feelings of anxiety as it is known to help regulate the heartbeat. Low levels of potassium may cause symptoms like heart palpitations, which produce a sensation that is commonly linked to stress or anxiety. However, in some cases this really is a sign of a nutritional deficiency.[24]

Avocados also improve the bioavailability of nutrients. In other words, when you eat avocado, your body is better able to absorb more of certain nutrients from other foods and supplements.[25]

Ways of Incorporating Avocado in Your Anxiety-Free Kitchen

- Eat an avocado whole, as a snack; just scoop it out with a spoon. You can add a squeeze of lemon and sprinkle some broccoli sprouts, hempseeds, or sesame seeds on top, or just eat it plain.

- When you serve soup, add some cubed avocado; it makes a great nutrient booster and adds a nice, creamy texture.

- Avocado can make smoothies super creamy and smooth.

- Did you know you can freeze avocado? Some juice bars freeze it in little cubes so it can be added as a healthy fat booster to whatever they're blending up.

- You can use avocado oil for a bread dip when you're entertaining. It has a delicious flavor on its own or you can season it.

- You can make any epic salad dressing with avocado oil as a base.

- Use avocado as a spread instead of butter, cream cheese, mayonnaise, etc.

Anxiety-Free Recipes with Avocado

- Grounding Lentil Soup with Avocado and Ginger
- Guacamole Greens Salad
- Brain Bowl with Walnut Pesto Sauce
- Chocolate Avocado Mousse

#6 OLIVE OIL

Olive oil made from European olives (*Olea europaea*) grown in the Mediterranean region is full of vitamins and other nutrients. Extra-virgin olive oil, which is derived from the first pressing of the olives, has the most delicate flavor and most potent antioxidant benefits.

The nutritional composition of olive oil is complex. Rich in MUFAs, it is composed mainly of mixed triglyceride esters of oleic acid, palmitic acid, and other fatty acids; traces of squalene and sterols; and other antioxidants—tyrosol, hydroxytyrosol, oleocanthal, oleuropein (OLE), vitamin E, and carotenoids.

OLE prevents the oxidation of LDL (aka "bad cholesterol") particles.[26] Everybody knows we are supposed to keep our bad cholesterol in check and raise our good cholesterol (HDL) if we can. But where this LDL-limiting trait becomes relevant to anxiety is in the ability of OLE to reduce anxiety-like responses by activating neurons that regulate the neurotransmitter serotonin and some neuropeptides. Neuropeptides help the neurons communicate with each other. They are signaling molecules that influence the activity of the brain and the body in specific ways. In one study, daily OLE administration was demonstrated to significantly reduce anxiety. Among other things it did, OLE blocked a stress-induced decrease in serotonin. This finding suggests that OLE has anxiolytic-like effects that could be helpful to people with PTSD and anxiety.[27]

Researchers have also looked into whether olive oil can modulate the serotonin, dopamine, norepinephrine, epinephrine, and/or histamine neurotransmitter systems in the brain. Neurochemical results show that repeated administration of olive oil decreases levels of 5-hydroxytryptamine (5-HT), 5-hydroxyindoleacetic acid (5-HIAA), and L-dopa and increases homovalinic acid (HVA). These findings suggest that olive oil has neuroprotective effects and reduces certain metabolically linked behavioral deficits. The researchers concluded that olive oil "could be used as a therapeutic substance for the treatment of depression and anxiety."[28]

Olive oil is rich in both omega-3 and omega-6 fatty acids and helps to balance them in the body. It supports the central nervous system by aiding proper nerve function and increasing serotonin levels. This gives it therapeutic value for treating major depression.[29]

Olive oil also could play an adaptive role in stressful times, as it has been shown to reduce even the perception of stress.[30]

Also, oleuropein derivatives found in olive oil, especially hydroxytyrosol, have been shown to have an antioxidant capacity higher than that of other known antioxidants, including vitamins E and C.[31]

Ways of Incorporating Olive Oil in Your Anxiety-Free Kitchen

- Olive oil has a medium smoke point, so use it for cooking foods at medium heat like stir-fried vegetables.

- Use olive oil as a base for salad dressing. You can't go wrong by mixing olive oil and a vinegar, like apple cider vinegar, for a delicious dressing, or olive oil and lemon.

- If you don't like the taste of olive oil, consider chopping up the leaves and tossing them into a salad, or making stuffed grape leaves like they do in Mediterranean countries. (The leaves of the olive tree have long been used in folk healing in France, Greece, Italy, Morocco, Spain, Tunisia, and Turkey.[32] Olive leaves have been used in the human diet in the form of extracts, herbal teas, and powders for centuries.)

Anxiety-Free Recipes with Olive Oil

- Basic Salad Dressing
- Green Sprout Salad
- Guacamole Greens Salad
- Grounding Lentil Soup with Avocado and Ginger

#7 COCONUT OIL

Coconut oil is anxiolytic. Virgin coconut oil, which may be produced from fresh coconut meat, coconut milk, or coconut milk residue, is rich in medium-chain triglycerides (MCTs), polyphenols, and lauric acid. Because of its nutritional chemistry, coconut oil is known to help protect us from the effects of stress on our bodies and reduce depression and anxiety.

Coconut oil is a *functional food*. I like this definition from the Mayo Clinic: "Functional foods are foods that have a positive effect on health beyond basic nutrition."[33] There was a study of rodents put under stress that were treated with virgin coconut oil. These subjects were found to exhibit higher levels of brain antioxidants, lower levels of brain 5-HT, and reduced weight of the adrenal glands compared to the control group. Serum cholesterol, triglyceride, glucose, and corticosterone levels were also lower. These researchers concluded: "The measure suggests that virgin coconut oil has value as an anti-stress functional oil."[34]

Due to the inflammatory nature of multiple sclerosis (MS), the disease increases anxiety levels for people who have it. A study was done to ascertain if coconut oil and green tea put together could help lessen the anxiety within this population. Green tea is laden with the polyphenol epigallocatechin gallate (EGCG), which has been studied intensively. This particular study was conducted for four months with 51 MS patients who received 800 milligrams of EGCG and 60 milliliters of coconut oil per day. Their state anxiety (how you feel in any moment) and trait anxiety (how you feel generally) were assessed before and after the study. The researchers concluded that coconut oil and EGCG were effective together in lessening anxiety.[35]

Please don't be afraid of the fats in coconut oil. It's full of good fats that we need to be healthy. Also, if you look at members of societies that live off coconut, they are not overweight. Good fats from coconut oil will not make you overweight. Hopefully, you understand by now (or are at least beginning to grasp) that it is processed foods, like refined sugar and carbs, that make us overweight and unhealthy.

Coconut oil combined with exercise was shown in another study to ameliorate the effects of stress on anxiety. Researchers concluded that coconut oil can be especially helpful during the critical period of brain development.[36] So many children and young people today feel anxious about what's happening in our world—everything from the pandemic to social media bullying and worrying about whether they'll be able to find work after school. I can't help but wonder what this is doing to their brains. If coconut oil can help, then it may be worth adding to the diet.

Ways of Incorporating Coconut Oil in Your Anxiety-Free Kitchen

- Use coconut oil for cooking. It has a higher smoke point than olive oil, so it's great for frying and baking.

- Use coconut oil as a base for salad dressing. Try a liquid coconut oil, like an MCT oil, that doesn't need to be melted.

- If you don't like the smell or taste of coconut oil, I understand. A lot of people don't! If this is the case, you can opt for a "refined" coconut oil, which means it's gone through an extra process to remove the smell and taste of coconut. It's still healthy. I use this kind of coconut oil in my dessert recipes to make cookies, cakes, cashew ice cream, and cashew cheesecake because I want the coconut oil health benefits and consistency, but don't want the smell or flavor.

- Use the butter-flavored coconut oil as a replacement for dairy butter. (I recommend Nutiva brand.) It smells and tastes like butter, making it a great butter alternative, but it's made from coconut oil, so it's healthier!

Anxiety-Free Recipes with Coconut Oil

- Master Smoothie
- Chicken Noodle Soup
- Mini Cashew Cheesecakes
- Ice Cream Bites with Chocolate Sauce

#8 BROCCOLI AND BROCCOLI SPROUTS

Broccoli and broccoli sprouts both have so many amazing compounds that can help us reduce our anxiety. Perhaps their most powerful and studied component is sulforaphane—basically a sulfur-rich compound. A full-grown head of broccoli does contain sulforaphane, but broccoli sprouts have 10 to 100 times more! On day three or four of growing broccoli, when the sprouts are one to two inches tall, this is when the sulforaphane is highest. According to a report published in the *Proceedings of the National Academy of Sciences*, just a small one-ounce serving provides 73 milligrams of sulforaphane glucosinolate. Per 100-gram serving, broccoli sprouts offer approximately 250 milligrams.[37]

A group of scientists from major medical centers in the United States reports: "There is robust epidemiological evidence for the beneficial effects of broccoli consumption on brain health, many of them clearly mediated by the isothiocyanate sulforaphane it contains—since first isolated from broccoli and demonstrated to have chemoprotective properties in the early 1990s, over 3,000 publications have described its efficacy."[38] Nonetheless, they don't conclude that there is a definitive quantity of broccoli to eat—a magic portion size—to gain neuroprotective benefits, so we should simply plan to eat it frequently. I personally eat broccoli sprouts every few days to ensure I am getting some sulforaphane into my cells.

I wrote a lot about broccoli and broccoli sprouts in my book *Cancer-Free with Food*, because it's an incredible ingredient. Many of the nutritional compounds that make it an anticancer blockbuster will help you feel better if you have anxiety, too. Broccoli is a cruciferous vegetable known to be a rich source of glucosinolates, flavonoids, vitamins C and E, and minerals.[39] In particular, the isothiocyanates and indole derivatives in it, including sulforaphane, phenylethyl isothiocyanate, and indole-3-carbinol, are reported to induce antioxidant activities.[40]

During oxidative stress, large amounts of reactive oxygen species such as hydrogen peroxide (H_2O_2), hydroxyl radical, and superoxide anion are produced that damage DNA. DNA damage leads to mutations that, in turn, are associated with diseases such as cancer and coronary heart disease, as well as inflammatory diseases such as arteriosclerosis and anxiety disorders.[41] We know that anti-inflammatory foods such as broccoli help to inhibit oxidative stress. Broccoli is a powerful anti-inflammatory and, no doubt, amazing brain food.

Ways of Incorporating Broccoli in Your Anxiety-Free Kitchen

- Steam, bake, or fry your broccoli. Fry it in some avocado oil with a high smoke point or bake it with some coconut oil and sea salt. Absolutely delicious.

- Whenever you make soups or stir-fried vegetables, always think to add broccoli to your dish. It also goes well as a side with salmon and meat dishes.

- Shave some broccoli into your scrambled eggs or omelet. You can also shave it and add it to a salad.

- I use a greens powder that has broccoli and broccoli sprouts in it. I mix this with water almost daily. You can add broccoli powder to juices, shakes, and smoothies as well.

- Chop the broccoli and add it to a salad. Sulforaphane is produced largely from glucoraphanin during the chopping or crushing of broccoli.[42]

Ways of Incorporating Broccoli Sprouts in Your Anxiety-Free Kitchen

- You can purchase broccoli sprouts at many health food stores and certain grocery stores. Broccoli sprouts have a shorter shelf life and cost more than other types of sprouts, so not every supermarket carries them. It is easy to grow your own, though, and you can watch online videos for guidance on this.

- Start to think of broccoli sprouts as a kitchen staple. Stock up on some every week, and then think, *How can I add broccoli sprouts to this?* whenever you're cooking. Add them to everything from soups and salads to main dishes. Sprinkle them on meats or place a wild salmon fillet on a plate full of sprouts. Daily intake of broccoli sprouts also normalizes bowel habits in healthy human subjects.[43]

- Roll up broccoli sprouts into balls and add them to ice cube trays with water. Then pop a few of these into your smoothies and shakes! Freeze a bunch of them so you always have them on hand ready to add. This idea came from my friend Doug Evans, who wrote *The Sprout Book*.

Anxiety-Free Recipes with Broccoli

- Broccoli Popcorn
- Stir-Fried Satay Noodles
- Rainbow Veggie Stir-Fry
- Brain Bowl with Walnut Pesto Sauce

Anxiety-Free Recipes with Broccoli Sprouts

- Super Greens Juice
- Brain Bowl with Walnut Pesto Sauce
- Green Sprout Salad
- Walnut-Crusted Chicken Salad

#9 GINGER

The amazing and almighty ginger! Ginger is a root vegetable that is well-recognized as a form of herbal medicine. It is a member of the same plant family as cardamom and turmeric.

Ginger has benefits beyond flavoring your favorite stir-fry recipe or easing an upset stomach. Animal studies have indicated that it can raise serotonin levels and, therefore, may treat and reduce anxiety as successfully as benzodiazepine drugs![44] We know that serotonin is manufactured in the gut, and ginger is commonly used to ease an upset stomach.

In fact, ginger is purported to have a variety of powerful therapeutic and preventive benefits. There is clear evidence of the effectiveness of ginger as an antioxidant, anti-inflammatory agent. It also may be helpful for treating nausea and cancer. Ginger is known to decrease markers of age-related oxidative stress, such as inflammation, swelling, and pain, and has been used for thousands of years for the treatment of hundreds of ailments like these.

With its delightfully tangy and invigorating scent and flavor, ginger is one of the most commonly consumed dietary condiments in the world. The resin from its rhizomes (roots) contains many bioactive components, which is why this pungent ingredient is believed to produce a variety of remarkable pharmacological and physiological effects. Interest in ginger as an effective preventive and its therapeutic agents has increased significantly in recent years. It is being studied alongside turmeric and black pepper— with which it forms a kind of triumvirate ingredient in Indian cuisine, which is famously anti-inflammatory. From scientific studies, we now know that ginger exerts its anti-inflammatory power by suppressing the action of COX-2, the enzyme responsible for swelling and pain, and inhibiting the biosynthesis of the inflammatory mediators prostaglandin and leukotriene.[45]

According to several valid and reliable studies I have read that date back to the 1990s, the anxiolytic activity of ginger is very real.[46]

Caution: Although ginger is considered to be safe, if you are on any medications, please check with your doctor that it will be okay for you and is not contraindicated by medications you are taking.

Ways of Incorporating Ginger in Your Anxiety-Free Kitchen

- Cut it up and boil it to make ginger tea.
- Juice it and add it to smoothies.
- Put a few drops of ginger essential oil or ginger extract in your stir-fry near the end of cooking.

Anxiety-Free Recipes with Ginger

- Super Greens Juice
- Hotshot Citrus
- Anti-Inflammatory Ginger Tea
- Thai Chicken Pizza

#10 Cacao

Cacao is remarkably high in magnesium—it has 40 times more than blueberries! The cacao bean is chocolate in its natural state before it's heat-processed to become cocoa and then chocolate.

All of the chocolate I make at home is made with cacao powder, including the recipes in this book. In my previous book, cacao was featured as #9 on the list of anticancer foods due to studies proving it to have antitumor effects and the ability to help prevent brain cancer! Cacao releases those feel-good emotions in the body and brain. It also is an excellent source of good, healthy fats.

Cacao improves our mood almost instantly. Even just the smell of it can activate feel-good brain chemicals and influence brain activity in a positive manner! An experiment was done of human subjects in which researchers found that the aroma of chocolate was associated with deep relaxation.[47]

There have been countless studies on cacao—as well as cocoa and dark chocolate—proving that it helps to reduce anxiety, stress, depression, and inflammation. Cacao is one of the richest sources of flavanol antioxidants on earth! Flavonoid-rich chocolate can enhance the endogenous antioxidant activities of the body, resulting in reduced oxidative damage.[48]

In one study, changes in self-reported anxiety and other undesirable emotional and energetic states were recorded as a function of having eaten chocolate just after consumption and up to one hour later![49] Another study showed that daily consumption of milk or dark chocolate for just two weeks reduced perceived stress in subjects. (White chocolate, which does not contain flavonoid-rich cocoa solids, did not have the same effect on the subjects.)[50] It's no wonder we crave chocolate, and no wonder we feel better when we eat it!

Cacao polyphenols have been shown to reduce stress in the highly stressed, as well as in "normal healthy" individuals, especially women. In the study described above, it was observed that gender-specific differences in perceived stress scores following chocolate intake possibly could be partly attributed to the effects of female sex hormones.[51]

Scientific evidence shows that the hypothalamic-pituitary-adrenal axis response during stressful events differs markedly between men and women. There is an increased sensitivity of the adrenal cortex in women as compared to men. As you may be aware, the adrenal glands produce hormones that trigger the fight-or-flight response throughout the sympathetic nervous system. They make us anxious so that we can handle danger. Where this goes awry for too many of us, and becomes uncomfortable, is when this response is triggered when no danger is present, or if we cannot settle down again once the danger has passed.

The neuroprotective effects of cacao and its influence on cognitive performance can be attributed to its widespread stimulation of blood flow to the brain. Its antioxidant molecules, mainly flavonoids like epicatechin (think dark chocolate and green tea), are responsible. It's beneficial to eat dark chocolate on days when you know you are going to be under stress, such as the day of an exam at school or a presentation or long workday at the office—even on your wedding day. The flavonoids in chocolate induce positive moods.

In addition, flavonoids signal cascades of brain chemicals to be released that inhibit the death of brain cells—thus, reducing anxiety. The cacao bean is one of the most concentrated sources of theobromine, which is a methylxanthine similar to caffeine. But unlike caffeine, which is extremely stimulating, theobromine has only a mild stimulatory effect on the central nervous system. Cacao is also a good source of several other compounds with biological activity, biogenic amines (neurotransmitters) such as serotonin, tryptophan, tyrosine, tryptamine, tyramine, and phenylethylamine.[52]

Balancing the gut is a strategy for improving the balance of neurotransmitters and improving vitamin absorption. One study of the effects of cacao on gut health and metabolism found it to be helpful. Consuming dark chocolate reduced the stress hormones cortisol and catecholamine, and it partially normalized stress-related differences in energy metabolism. The study provides strong evidence that daily consumption of 40 grams of dark chocolate over a period of two weeks is sufficient.[53] That's roughly one and a half ounces, so just a couple squares of a high-quality dark chocolate would do it. Eat up!

Consumption of cocoa flavanols results in acute improvements in mood and cognitive performance during sustained mental effort. A study investigated what would happen during sustained mental demand, using consumption of cacao drinks. Increases in self-reported "mental fatigue" were significantly reduced by the consumption of the beverage. It is suggested that this may be related to the effects of cacao on endothelial function and blood flow.[54]

What's stopping us from reaping the benefits of cacao? Unfortunately, most people think chocolate is unhealthy because they equate it with sweets and believe sweets are bad for us. As a result, they try to suppress their cravings for chocolate. In reality, the health issues associated with chocolate come from the white sugar, poor-quality dairy, and soy lecithin used to make most poor-quality chocolate. That type of chocolate will do damage, and, in fact, can increase our anxiety because of the other ingredients mixed with the cacao. High-quality chocolate, however, can heal and restore us. Some chocolate dishes are even savory—think of the mole sauce in traditional Mexican cuisine. It's an elixir of yummy goodness.

Don't worry about gaining weight with chocolate; eating it can actually do the opposite! I lost weight by eating organic chocolate sweetened without refined sugar every day. We are more likely to gain weight from consuming refined sugar and dairy. A 2012 study concluded that frequent chocolate consumption is actually associated with a lower body mass index.[55]

Trust your gut instincts to discern if cacao is the right healing food for you. And also keep track of how you feel right after eating it, then an hour later, and even up through the next day. (Handle tomatoes, mushrooms, and lentils the same way; they can be healing for some but are poison for others.) Cacao beans contain low variable amounts of caffeine, a well-known psychostimulant, meaning it stimulates the central nervous system. Avoid it if it makes you feel terrible.

Ways of Incorporating Cacao
in Your Anxiety-Free Kitchen

- Add cacao powder to smoothies and shakes.
- Add cacao to a plant-based milk to make a chocolate milk.
- Add cacao to hot water to make a hot chocolate.
- Make homemade chocolate recipes using cacao.

Anxiety-Free Recipes with Cacao

- Chocolate Supreme Smoothie
- Hot Chocolate
- Moist Chocolate SunButter Brownies
- Chocolate Sauce–Covered Strawberries

OTHER AMAZING ANXIETY-FREE FOODS WORTH NOTING

Here are a few more ingredients you will want to incorporate into your diet if you're anxious.

Strawberries

Strawberries provide a rich amount of antioxidants, which anyone with anxiety needs more of, particularly vitamin C. In fact, strawberries made #14 on the berries, fruit, and vegetable analyses in the Antioxidant Food Table. Multiple studies have shown that a diet rich in vitamin C may improve mood, support healthy brain function, help calm you, and put you in a better frame of mind.

Why else do strawberries make us feel happy? I think it's because the folate in strawberries lowers the homocysteine level in our bloodstreams. Unhealthy amounts of the amino acid homocysteine prevent our glands from producing dopamine and serotonin, hormones associated with happiness.[56] That leads to us feeling anxious and sad. Strawberries prevent homocysteine from forming in unhealthy amounts, and therefore they enable the blood to deliver these important chemicals to the brain.

A strawberry looks like a heart. When we eat a strawberry, it gives us a psychological reminder that we are receiving love and strengthening our heart—and the more love we experience, the less anxiety we will have. Doesn't looking at a fresh, juicy red strawberry just make you so happy?

There is a risk that strawberries may contain pesticide residue, so it is important to buy organic strawberries or grow your own! They are worth the effort, as your antioxidant levels will increase just half an hour after eating these delicious beauties.

Anxiety-Free with Food Recipes with Strawberries

- Strawberry Milkshake
- Chocolate Tigernut Berry Smoothie
- Brain Bowl
- Chocolate Sauce–Covered Strawberries

Oranges

Isn't it interesting that when we get a cold or feel our immunity is running low, we often crave oranges? Oranges contain vitamin C and a lot of other antioxidants, so you definitely want them in your fruit bowl. They are so cheerful, even just looking at a vibrant orange can brighten our mood. But combined with their scent and flavor, well, the impact is incomparable. As we saw with chocolate, odors are capable of altering our emotional states! So, enjoy peeling your orange and breathe in its scent as much as you can!

I would also recommend sniffing some orange essential oil (which is distilled from the juice of orange peels) straight out of the bottle or putting it in your diffuser.

Anxiety-Free with Food Recipes with Oranges

- Vitamin C Blast
- Hotshot Citrus
- Rainbow Veggie Stir-Fry
- Chocolate-Dipped Oranges with Roasted Hazelnuts and Walnuts

* * *

- **Pineapple:** Pineapple not only helps improve digestion because of the enzymes it contains but also reduces depression and anxiety. Perhaps this is due to the fact that the fruit offers us the amino acid tryptophan, which supports production of serotonin.

- **Other fruits:** Bananas, apples, grapefruit, lemons, blackberries, cucumbers, kiwifruit, and blueberries should be included in your eating plan for anxiety because of their high nutrient content.

- **Other great seeds:** Prepare meals with chia seeds, hempseeds, flaxseeds, sunflower seeds, and pumpkin seeds. Sunflower seeds were #3 on the analysis of nuts, legumes, and grain products in the Antioxidant Food Table. Sesame seeds also contain great levels of zinc, which is often touted as a supplement for anxiety.[57]

- **Other great nuts:** Snack on Brazil nuts, cashews, almonds, and pecans, or include them in your prepared dishes. Pecans were #2 on the analysis of nuts, legumes, and grains in the Antioxidant Food Table.[58]

- **Other great vegetables:** Asparagus is a rich source of tryptophan (a serotonin aid). Shiitake mushrooms are high in vitamin C.

- **Oats:** Oats are incredibly calming—I consider them a comfort food. Multiple studies show that they have mild antidepressant effects, increase our ability to cope with stress, are anti-inflammatory, and reduce anxiety.[59] In a study conducted at the Nutritional Physiology Research Centre at the University of South Australia, Adelaide, a dose of 2,500 milligrams of an extract of wild oats significantly increased brain activity in the left frontotemporal region of participants during a concentration task two hours after supplementation![60] In addition, oats contain unique bioactive phytochemical compounds known as avenanthramides, which have strong anti-inflammatory properties.[61] See my Brainiac Porridge recipe (p. 175) for a soothing breakfast with antianxiety toppings.

- **Other meats to eat in moderation:** Turkey is the classic source of tryptophan. Also include eggs and oysters (which contain zinc and copper) in your meal plan.

Nine Drinks That Calm

- Green tea. This powerful drink contains a brain-relaxing compound called theanine to reduce anxiety.

- Water

- Fresh green juice

- Fresh vegetable juice

- Chamomile tea

- Valerian tea. This medicinal herb—often found in bedtime tea blends—has been credited with reducing nervousness, anxiety, and insomnia.

- Cherry juice with no added sugar

- Black tea

- Genius Smoothie (p. 158)

CHAPTER 3

Top Antianxiety Supplements

Tackling the problem of anxiety with supplements can be a powerful solution. Based on the available evidence, it appears that nutritional and herbal supplementation is an incredibly effective method for treating anxiety and anxiety-related conditions, usually without the risk of serious side effects. In fact, many supplements have been proven even more effective than some conventional medications.[1]

The supplements I recommend in this chapter are natural, made either using ingredients that come from nature or straight from foods. A lot of these supplements are anxiolytic as well as immune boosting. There is evidence that too much anxiety can weaken the immune system dramatically. Anxiety puts stress on the body, which, in turn, releases cortisol that creates more anxiety in the body. Anxiety is a two-way street. We also know that people who are unwell tend to feel more anxiety. The biologic effects of stress on immunity are multifaceted, including complex neuroendocrine and neurotransmitter interactions.[2] Neuroendocrine cells receive messages from nerves and respond by releasing hormones into the bloodstream. Hormones coordinate and influence metabolic functions, mood, and behavior.

Why We Need a Boost of Nutrients

A supplement is either a pill, capsule, tablet, powder, or liquid that is designed to complement a diet of whole and prepared foods and beverages by providing missing nutrients or extra doses of certain nutrients. Supplements can be incredibly useful for rapidly putting sufficient amounts of a nutrient into your body, especially if you are nutrient deficient.

Nutrient absorption can vary from person to person, even meal to meal. The number of nutrients that your body absorbs from food as you metabolize it in the digestive tract can range from less than 10 percent to greater than 90 percent. Adequate nutrient levels are vital to our well-being and yet there are many possible causes for poor nutrient absorption: having a weak gut lining; a microbiome imbalance, such as a bacterial or fungal overgrowth (aka dysbiosis); damage to the intestines from inflammation or infection; prolonged use of antibiotics; celiac disease; leaky gut syndrome; Crohn's disease; food allergies; surgery; liver disease; pancreatic insufficiency; or an autoimmune disease.

After years of junk-food binge eating, I had done so much damage to my gut that I was not absorbing nutrients from the majority of what I ate. Although I was eating a lot of food, I was chronically malnourished! My solution was to do a detoxifying cleanse and follow this up with supplementation to boost my nutrient intake. Clean, whole foods are the ideal source of nutrition if you are healthy and your organs are functioning well. But in my opinion, doing a detox is incredibly important if you are unwell and you want to ensure that your body is absorbing the maximum quantity of nutrients from your foods and supplements.

Note: We have to be careful when choosing supplements because some of the manufacturers in the supplement industry are sneaky with their ingredients—they dilute or replace them—and some will manufacture a substandard product that costs very little to make while charging a huge price for it.

It is important to make sure you read the ingredient labels, as some contain fillers, additives, colors, and synthetics. A plant-based vegetarian outer capsule is best. Once you get to know the supplement brands you can trust, stick to them.

While researching this book, the studies were so compelling that I immediately started taking many of these supplements. However, I was so concerned about quality, I was moved to offer my own Anxiety-Free daily support supplement! I was involved in every step of the process, so I know every ingredient is high quality. I personally take these supplements them every day. You'll find my recommendations for trusted brands, as well as information about the supplements I created, in the Resources and LianaWernerGray.com/AnxietyFree.

RESPECTING YOUR BIOINDIVIDUALITY

It might come as a relief to you to know there are many great supplements that can help reduce anxiety—some providing noticeable differences within *minutes* of taking them. I was immediately excited when researching this topic.

It's important to mention that I do not take *all* the supplements in this chapter, nor do I recommend that you do so! I wanted to provide you with a comprehensive list, so I've included the most common supplements, those with the best scientific backing, and my personal favorites so you could decide for yourself which supplements would be best for you.

Here is where the principle of bioindividuality comes into play. It is an invitation for you to choose the foods and supplements that work for you and your unique needs rather than what's considered "best." I recommend introducing supplements slowly, one at a time, so you can tune in to your body and really feel what each one is doing. Remember to read labels carefully to figure out doses and any contraindications. Be sure to ask the advice of your doctor or health-care professional before taking supplements, especially if you are taking any medications or have health conditions. There are many supplements that can affect pharmaceuticals that a person is taking. Now let's jump into an A-to-Z guide to the most recommended and studied antianxiety supplements.

The A-to-Z Guide to Antianxiety Supplements

- Açai

- Aloe vera/aloe juice

- Amino acids

- Arginine, see Amino acids

- Ashwagandha

- Astragalus

- B-complex vitamins

- Blue-green algae (Cyanobacteria)

- Burdock root

- Cannabinoidal (CBD) oil

- Cannabis (marijuana/THC)

- Chamomile

- Chlorella, see Blue-green algae

- Chlorophyll

- Copper, colloidal

- Curcumin, see Turmeric

- Essential oils

- Fish oil, see Omega-3 fatty acids

- Folate, see B-complex vitamins

- GABA (gamma-aminobutyric acid)

- Gold, colloidal

- Holy basil (tulsi)

- Inositol, see B-complex vitamins

- Kava kava

- Lemon balm

- Licorice root

- Lysine, see Amino acids

- Magnesium

- Melatonin

- Niacin (vitamin B$_3$), see B-complex vitamins

- Omega-3 fatty acids

- Passionflower

- Prebiotics

- Probiotics

- Rhodiola

- Schisandra, or Schizandra

- Silver, colloidal

- Spirulina, see Blue-green algae

- St. John's wort

- Theanine, see Amino acids

- Thiamine, see B-complex vitamins

- Tryptophan, see Amino acids

- Tulsi, see Holy basil

- Turmeric

- Tyrosine, see Amino acids

- Zinc

Açai

Açai berries are a superfood because of their antioxidant and anti-inflammatory potency, which comes from being high in polyphenols. By reducing intestinal inflammation, they help secure the gut-brain relationship.[3] Countless studies have shown that açai is an antidepressant and neuroprotective—it helps preserve neuronal structure and function.[4] *Neurons* are brain cells.

In Part II, "Anxiety-Free with Food Recipes," you'll find an epic Açai Bowl recipe (see p. 180). To supplement with açai, you take it in powdered form in capsules. For the correct dosage on these, follow the packaging instructions.

Aloe Vera/Aloe Juice

Aloe vera is a gelatinous substance obtained from a succulent plant that grows in tropical climates. It has been suggested that it has antidiabetic, antioxidative, and—more important for those experiencing anxiety—neuroprotective effects. There is a chemical mechanism in aloe that protects neurons in the hippocampus, a brain structure embedded in the temporal lobe of the cerebral cortex that participates in regulating motivation, emotion, memory, and learning.[5] Research shows it improves behavioral deficits associated with anxiety, such as lethargy, poor concentration, and memory difficulties.

You can harvest pulp directly from an aloe plant yourself and blend it to make it a drinkable liquid, or buy fresh aloe juice from a store. Fresh blended is ideal. To the best of my knowledge, there is only one aloe company in the United States that sells raw and unfiltered aloe juice, which is flash-frozen when it is fresh and packaged without preservatives, Aloe 1 (see Resources for ordering details). You want pure aloe with no preservatives or anything else added. Aloe juice sold in supermarkets and organic food stores typically contains some preservatives to make it shelf-stable.

Aloe and Colloidal Silver Protocol

The aloe and silver protocol is used to cleanse the digestive tract (gut), reduce inflammation, boost immunity, and promote healthy gut microflora. I have found this to be the most successful cleanse protocol for my digestive system to date. Cleansing the gut reduces symptoms of anxiety by relieving intestinal distress and influencing the balance of good bacteria in the microbiome. The protocol is as follows:

- Drink 1 ounce of aloe vera and 1 ounce of colloidal silver (mixed together), 3 times a day on an empty stomach (morning, noon, and night). Eat 45 minutes later. Do this for 2 to 8 weeks. If you absolutely cannot drink the aloe juice because you do not like the taste, add it to coconut water or a Super Greens Juice (see p. 153) to mask the flavor.

- Take 1 dose of probiotics (see p. 95) before bed.

This cleansing protocol makes me feel hydrated, energized, refreshed, and alive. I learned to do this when I wanted my digestive system to be "squeaky clean" of parasites and bacteria; to repair any leaks in my intestinal walls; and to get rid of excess candida, bloating, and a sensation of heaviness I often felt in a certain area of my gut. Even the first time I did it, I found it soothing and enjoyable, and I experienced no detox symptoms from it at all. I have done this cleanse for three weeks, once a year, ever since then to refresh my digestive tract. Gut health has a powerful impact on the brain, for better or for worse, because of the neurotransmitters that are manufactured in the gut.

Amino Acids

Amino acids are the chemical building blocks of life. Both plants and animals make protein from these 20 precious substances. Amino acids that cannot be made inside the body are known as *essential amino acids*. These include histidine, isoleucine, leucine, lysine, methionine, phenylalanine, threonine, tryptophan, and valine. The amino acids that are particularly interesting in regard to reduction of anxiety are arginine, lysine, theanine, tryptophan, and tyrosine. If you're deficient in these or a neurochemical that is built from any of these amino acids, then supplementation may be helpful. For example, supplementing with amino acids is a great way of boosting your levels of GABA, a calming neurotransmitter.

Note: Sometimes you'll see an L in front of the name of the amino acid on supplement labels, which just means it is being provided in a form that is absorbable by the gut.

- *Arginine.* Arginine is found in red meat, poultry, fish, dairy products, nuts, seeds, legumes, and seaweed. It plays an important role in the treatment of heart disease due to its ability to block arterial plaque buildup, blood clots, and platelet clumping, and to increase blood flow through the coronary artery, which can help to ease anxiety as that affects blood flow. A study confirmed that supplementing the diet with a combination of lysine and arginine (both are amino acids) can be a useful dietary intervention in otherwise healthy humans with high subjective levels of mental stress and anxiety.[6]

  Arginine also can help relieve migraine headaches. It seems to be effective when taken along with the painkiller ibuprofen—starting to work within 30 minutes.[7]

  In addition, it can promote weight loss because it reduces fat mass and increases muscle mass by increasing the activity of insulin, which helps metabolize fats. Furthermore, arginine increases strength for exercise, thus making it doubly effective in a weight-loss program.[8]

- *Lysine.* Supplements of lysine are known to help balance levels of the hormone cortisol that rise when triggered by stress in both healthy individuals and those with high anxiety. Lysine is an amino acid used to make medicine for the prevention and treatment of cold sores caused by the herpes simplex labialis virus. Studies have identified that a diet fortified with lysine and arginine reduces plasma cortisol.[9] It has long been claimed by neuroscientists that the dysregulation of neurotransmitters, such as GABA, serotonin, dopamine, and norepinephrine, is a cause of anxiety.[10] According to Medical News Today, serotonin helps regulate "mood and social behavior, appetite and digestion, sleep, memory, and sexual desire and function."[11]

Plant-based ingredients that are sources of lysine are avocados, beets, leeks, tomatoes, pears, green and red bell peppers, potatoes, soybeans, kidney beans, navy beans, black beans, chickpeas, lentils, edamame, pumpkin seeds, pistachios, cashews, macadamia nuts, quinoa, and buckwheat. Animal-based ingredients that include lysine are beef, pork, lamb, poultry, cheese, eggs, and certain fish, including cod and sardines.

You can get L-lysine supplements. Other supplements that provide lysine are spirulina, chlorella, fish oil, and fenugreek seed.

- *Theanine.* Theanine is an amino acid that modulates aspects of brain function in humans. Evidence from human electroencephalograph (EEG) studies proves it has a direct effect.[12] Notably, theanine significantly increases activity in the alpha frequency bandwidth of brainwaves, which indicates that it relaxes the mind—without inducing drowsiness. Data also indicated that theanine, when consumed at realistic dietary levels, has a significant effect on the general state of our mental alertness or arousal. (Alpha wave activity is associated with the kind of attention and awareness we experience during meditation—a positive mental state.)[13]

Results from a study of people with anxiety disorders or under psychological stress suggest that theanine administered at doses ranging from 200 to 400 milligrams per day for up to eight weeks is safe and produces stress-reducing effects for people with acute and chronic symptoms.[14]

Fun fact: Tea is the most widely consumed beverage in the world after water. Green and black tea leaves are an excellent source of theanine, which is why it is so good to drink tea in the hour before bed when you're winding down. If you're sensitive to caffeine, choose decaffeinated teas.

L-theanine supplements are available at many drugstores and health food shops.

- *Tryptophan.* Tryptophan is an important amino acid that creates niacin, which creates the neurotransmitter serotonin. The brain needs tryptophan to create serotonin. Tryptophan is found in most protein-based foods, including red meat, eggs, fish, poultry, almonds, sunflower seeds, pumpkin seeds, spirulina, sesame seeds, milk, and even oats, chickpeas, and cacao.

- *Tyrosine.* Tyrosine helps to increase your levels of the neurotransmitter dopamine, which regulates movement, motivation, arousal, reinforcement, and reward—in fact, it's hard to find life satisfactory without enough dopamine in the brain. It is a great energy booster and stress reliever, as well as an appetite suppressor.

  Tyrosine is found in many foods, especially in cheese, where it was first discovered. (In fact, *tyros* means "cheese" in Greek.)[15] Tyrosine can also be found in beef, pork, chicken, turkey, fish (including salmon and tuna), eggs, beans (including white beans), nuts (including peanuts and almonds), seeds (including pumpkin seeds, sesame seeds, soybeans, and lima beans), green peas, spinach, corn, kiwifruit, cacao, okra, white and sweet potatoes, avocados, bananas, oats, wild rice, and wheat. Think of high-protein foods and you're probably on the money.

Supplementing with tyrosine increases levels of adrenaline and norepinephrine as well. By helping increase the levels of these neurotransmitters, tyrosine may help improve our memory and our ability to perform under pressure.[16] It is also a precursor of hormones produced by the thyroid gland that are responsible for regulating metabolism.[17] In addition, it is a precursor of important brain chemicals that help nerve cells communicate, which regulates mood.[18]

The United Nations University recommends a daily intake of 11 milligrams of tyrosine per pound of body weight (25 milligrams per kilogram).[19] But tyrosine's greatest anti-stress effects have been observed when it's taken in doses of 45 to 68 milligrams per pound (100 to 150 milligrams per kilogram) of body weight about 60 minutes before a stressful event occurs—so this is a good supplement if you have to do a work presentation or give a speech and the prospect is making you nervous.[20]

Caution: Tyrosine may interfere with some medications. If you are taking thyroid medications or have an overactive thyroid, be cautious when supplementing with tyrosine.

ARGININE, SEE AMINO ACIDS

ASHWAGANDHA

Ashwagandha, aka Indian ginseng (*Withania somnifera*), is derived from the fruit or leaf of a shrub. The name refers to the smell of the root ("like a horse"). In Latin, the species name, *somnifera*, means "sleep inducing." Most ashwagandha is cultivated in India, Nepal, and China. This has been used for centuries to alleviate fatigue and improve general well-being. It has powerful antianxiety, antioxidant, and anti-inflammatory properties. It is also an adaptogen, which means it helps the body respond to stress. One study in which people took 300 mg twice daily of high-concentration ashwagandha root extract found that it "safely and effectively improves an individual's resistance towards stress and thereby improves self-assessed quality of life."[21]

You can buy ashwagandha in the form of a loose powder, a capsule, a leaf, or a leaf extract. I take the capsules, but also have loose powder in my cupboard, which I add to smoothies, shakes, soups, and hot water (to make a tea). Some people boil it in water with milk and butter or honey. You could also mix it with plant-based milk with some ghee, coconut oil, and honey.

ASTRAGALUS

Astragalus is famous for boosting immunity. A plant that belongs to the legume family, its root is used as an herbal remedy in traditional Chinese medicine to reinforce *qi* (life force energy) and aid in the growth of new tissue. When I consume it, I love visualizing how astragalus helps the body build new cells.

Research at the UCLA AIDS Institute investigated the ability of cycloastragenol (a compound extracted from astragalus) to inhibit the aging process of immune cells. Scientists found it had positive effects on the cells' response to viral infections. It appeared to increase production of telomerase, an enzyme that plays a key role in cell replication and protects cells from DNA damage.[22]

You can buy dried astragalus root and make tea by boiling it in hot water. Or you can purchase it in the form of a powder, a liquid extract, or a capsule. The powder or liquid can be added to smoothies, teas, and soups.

B-Complex Vitamins

Roughly 90 years of research demonstrates the relevance of dietary nutrients for mental health. Some of the earliest research studies on nutrients relevant to mental illness observed irritability and mood problems in people known to be deficient in the B vitamins![23]

B vitamins are important for making sure the body's cells are functioning properly. Not only do they maintain healthy brain cells, they also help the body convert food into energy, create new blood cells, and maintain healthy skin and other tissues. All B vitamins are powerful immune boosters.

There are eight B vitamins, which are known collectively as B-complex vitamins:

B_1: thiamine

B_7: biotin

B_2: riboflavin

B_8: inositol

B_3: niacin

B_9: folate

B_5: pantothenic acid

B_{12}: cobalamin

B_6: pyridoxine

You can get B vitamins from proteins such as meat, eggs, and dairy products, as well as from leafy green vegetables, beans, and peas. Many kinds of cereal and some breads have B vitamins added to them because they are so critical for health. Bananas contain high amounts of vitamins B_6 and B_{12}, as well as magnesium and potassium. Vitamin B_6 comes in protein-rich foods like turkey and beans, as well as potatoes and spinach. Supplementing with B_6 is one way to increase your levels of GABA. Vitamin B_{12} is found in the following foods, listed highest to lowest in terms of the amount they contain: clams, liver, trout, salmon, tuna, beef, yogurt, milk, ham, eggs, and chicken. Nutritional yeast also contains B vitamins.[24] B_{12} can work alone as well as in conjunction with other B vitamins to support many vital functions.

Some things that cause a lack of B vitamins are atrophic gastritis, a condition in which your stomach lining has thinned; the presence of significant amounts of alcohol in your body; pernicious anemia, which makes it especially hard for your body to absorb vitamin B_{12}; conditions that affect your small intestines, such as Crohn's disease, celiac disease, bacterial growth, or a parasite; and immune system disorders, such as Graves' disease or lupus.

If someone has a deficiency in vitamin B_{12}, weakness, fatigue, and anxiety are common symptoms. They occur because your body doesn't have enough B_{12} to make the red blood cells that transport oxygen throughout your body. Vegans and other types of vegetarians sometimes have trouble consuming enough B_{12}, since B_{12} is found only in animal products. Vegan foods that have B_{12} in them, like nutritional yeast, are deliberately fortified with the supplement.

If you aren't getting enough nutrients in your diet or you eat a majority fast-food and processed-food diet, the first supplements you should consider taking are those in the B complex. A meta-analysis of 12 trials studying B vitamin supplementation provided evidence for its benefit for stress, concluding that it is particularly helpful for populations at risk due to poor nutrient status or poor mood status.[25]

In a study with more than 200 people, 73 percent of participants had success with thiamine as they experienced a disappearance of most of their anxiety symptoms! The researchers state, "For anxiety, thiamine has been used successfully at doses of 250 milligrams per day to treat patients with anxiety disorders, including those manifesting symptoms like chronic fatigue, insomnia, nightmares, anorexia, nausea and vomiting, diarrhea or constipation, chest and abdominal pain, depression, aggression, and headaches."[26]

Bright yellow urine is common when taking a B-complex supplement, specifically due to B_2, riboflavin. In fact, *flavin* comes from the Latin root word *flavus*, which means "yellow." Many people wonder if they should stop taking B vitamins when urine is yellow, but don't ditch them yet—they're actually a vital part of maintaining your overall health.

I strongly recommend having your doctor test you to see if you are vitamin B deficient. You can buy B-complex supplements, which include all eight B vitamins, or individual B supplements.

BLUE-GREEN ALGAE (CYANOBACTERIA)

Blue-green algae are some of the most nutrient-dense foods on the planet. You can find blue-green algae, such as spirulina and chlorella, marketed under various product names. Algae are found in almost every terrestrial and aquatic habitat: oceans and freshwater ponds and lakes, damp soil, and moist rocks in the deserts—even in Antarctic rocks! This pervasive life-form owes its superfood status to its high concentrations of protein, vitamins, and minerals. Through photosynthesis, it turns sunlight into oxygen in water.[27]

WebMD reports that people use blue-green algae for boosting the immune system, improving memory and otherwise assisting with good brain health, increasing energy and metabolism, and improving digestion and bowel health.[28]

You can buy blue-green algae in loose powder or capsule form. As for dosage, read package labels. You need only a tiny amount— perhaps a teaspoon per day. Too much can cause diarrhea.

Most powders are dark green. The Blue Majik powder is the most magical, sparkly blue I have ever seen. For visual appeal, I sometimes use this vibrant product in raw vegan desserts. You can also sprinkle it on your oats or cereal or mix it into your smoothies. Check out the Genius Smoothie recipe (p. 158) that includes spirulina!

Chlorella is a blue-green algae containing linoleic acid (omega-6 fatty acid), chlorophyll, and a lot of nutrients, including antioxidants, that help to repair DNA. One six-week study gave a chlorella supplement to people who smoked cigarettes. Participants who received the supplement experienced a 44 percent increase in blood levels of vitamin C, a 16 percent increase in levels of vitamin E, and a significant decrease in DNA damage.[29]

You can buy chlorella in capsules, liquid, or loose powder. It makes a terrific addition to smoothies.

Spirulina has become known as a superfood because it is incredibly nutrient-dense. It's packed full of vitamins, including A, C, E, and a range of Bs, as well as a whole host of minerals, such as calcium, iron, magnesium, selenium, and zinc. Along with all these important nutrients, spirulina helps reduce anxiety because it contains omega-3 fatty acids and chlorophyll. It can help protect our cells and tissues from damage and increases healthy microflora in the gut.[30]

Civilizations as far back as the Aztecs in the 16th century (and most likely much earlier—that's just recorded history) have used spirulina as food.[31] Due to its high protein content, NASA has used spirulina as a dietary supplement for its astronauts during space missions.[32] While chlorella and spirulina both contain high amounts of protein, studies have indicated that some strains of spirulina can contain up to 10 percent more protein than chlorella and the protein found in spirulina is also very well absorbed by the body.[33]

You can take spirulina in a capsule form. Personally, I love to add a teaspoon of it to my smoothies. I enjoy the taste, and you don't add much, so the taste isn't overpowering.

Caution: Check with your doctor before consuming spirulina, as people with allergies to seafood, seaweed, and other sea vegetables may want to avoid it. If you have a thyroid condition, an autoimmune disorder, gout, kidney stones, or phenylketonuria (PKU), or are pregnant or nursing, spirulina may not be appropriate for you. It also can possibly interfere with blood-thinning medication.

Spirulina vs. Chlorella

Which is better? Both are forms of algae and among the most popular algae supplements on the market. Chlorella is higher in fat and calories. They have the same amount of carbs. Chlorella is way higher in vitamin A, omega-3 fatty acids, magnesium, iron, and zinc. Spirulina is higher in copper. For the most part, chlorella and spirulina have the same amount of protein; however, some strains of spirulina are said to have more protein than chlorella. In conclusion: The high levels of antioxidants and other vitamins present in chlorella give it a slight nutritional advantage over spirulina.

BURDOCK ROOT, AKA HAPPY MAJOR (*ARCTIUM LAPPA*)

In some countries, burdock root is used as a vegetable. As a supplement, the root is dried and powdered. The active ingredients it possesses have been found to reduce inflammation and promote circulation, and it appears to be a promising agent for the prevention and treatment of neurodegenerative disorders implicated with oxidative stress, including anxiety.[34]

You can buy burdock as tea, capsules, or liquid extract, or even the whole root.

CANNABIDIOL (CBD) OIL

Studies show that cannabidiol, or CBD, which is a nonpsychoactive compound in cannabis, and only one of many, has clinical value in treating some neuropsychiatric disorders, including epilepsy, anxiety, and schizophrenia.[35] Evidence points toward a calming effect from CBD in the central nervous system. Unlike the compound tetrahydrocannabinol (THC) found in cannabis, CBD promotes relaxation but does not alter consciousness or trigger a "high."

You can consume CBD oil with a vape, by putting a few drops under your tongue, by adding it to foods or juices, or through topical application (combining it with a lotion or carrier oil). People are enjoying it at bedtime to relieve stress and pain and to help them sleep. If you are concerned about blood testing in your place of employment, be alert when you're making your purchase. CBD does not usually contain THC; however, some CBD oil brands will contain 0.3 percent THC. This is said not to show up on a drug test and does not cause any psychoactive effects, but you must use your own due diligence.[36]

There have been studies that strongly support CBD oil as a treatment for generalized anxiety disorder, panic disorder, social anxiety disorder, obsessive-compulsive disorder, and post-traumatic stress disorder.[37]

Cannabis (Marijuana/THC)

Cannabis (aka marijuana) is a psychoactive natural remedy, which is not to everyone's liking. It has only recently become legal in parts of the United States—but be careful because it is still illegal on a federal level in the United States and in scores of countries around the world. Even if you are using it medicinally, you do not want to travel with it and risk arrest while crossing borders.

Many people are attracted to cannabis for the relief of pain, while others use it recreationally. There are hundreds of compounds found in the plant, including THC; the compounds chemically related to THC (including CBD) are called cannabinoids. Research on the use of cannabis to treat anxiety disorders have found mixed results. While many studies found strong evidence for the anxiolytic effects of marijuana, one researcher noted the risk of "rebound anxiety" if usage is stopped, thereby fostering a dependence on the substance. Some studies found short-term benefits but an increased risk of harm in the long term.[38]

I have personally known people who found great relief while using it, although others say it produces *more* anxiety and even paranoia for them. The varied results in taking cannabis medicinally truly speak to the importance of respecting one's bioindividuality—what works for me may not work for you!

If you do choose to use cannabis to reduce your anxiety, I recommend it not as a long-term strategy but for short-term relief. Adverse effects of smoking cannabis are different in chronic smokers as compared to those who smoke only occasionally. However, prolonged consumption of cannabis has been shown to induce pathological conditions that involve disturbances in emotion, such as irritability, heightened anxiety, and depression.[39]

Furthermore, smoking marijuana has been said to be quite toxic to the lungs. In addition to the heat, which can damage sensitive lung tissue, "Marijuana smoke contains polycyclic aromatic hydrocarbons and carcinogens at higher concentrations than tobacco smoke. Cellular, tissue, animal, and human studies, as well as epidemiological studies, show that marijuana smoke is a risk factor for lung cancer."[40] As a result of this disturbance to the tissues, the act of smoking may trigger an anxiety response from your lungs. If this has happened to you, you may want to ingest rather than smoke THC, for example through gummies or baked goods.

Chamomile

Chamomile tea can be effective in relaxing the mood and inducing sleep. You can also take chamomile in pill form, as an extract, or as an essential oil (see "Essential Oils"). Studies have been conducted that show chamomile has anxiolytic and antidepressant effects.[41] Chamomile tea also offers the great benefits of relaxing the muscles and reducing irritability.

Chlorella, see Blue-Green Algae

CHLOROPHYLL

My absolute favorite supplement in the world is chlorophyll—the green pigment in plants—and I wish every human being were consuming it on a daily basis. Chlorophyll is a compound found in dark leafy greens like kale, spinach, collard greens, dandelion greens, and turnip greens, broccoli and broccoli sprouts, and blue-green algae, like chlorella and spirulina. Although I feel that chlorophyll has been understudied, it has been shown to have many health benefits. This is one of the best health hacks we have available to us! A lot of high-performance people have discovered its value already.

It is noteworthy that chlorophyll contains magnesium, which we know helps to reduce anxiety. People with low magnesium intake are likely to experience anxiety. What are the other benefits? Chlorophyll reduces inflammation in the body. It has been shown to enhance oxidative stress tolerance, meaning that your body will be able to adapt to stressful conditions more easily. It also contains a lot of healthful antioxidants.[42]

Chlorophyll helps put fresh oxygen into the body, which gives us instant energy. The chemical structure of the molecule of chlorophyll in a plant is similar to the chemical structure of the molecule of hemoglobin in the human bloodstream, which carries oxygen to our cells. The difference is that chlorophyll is made up of magnesium rather than iron, like red blood cells. Chlorophyll also helps to prevent blood sugar from dropping, which can help stop us from impulsive eating when our sugar level is low.

Because chlorophyll has so many antianxiety properties, it should be consumed daily. Luckily, you consume chlorophyll every time you eat a green vegetable, have a leafy salad, or drink a Super Greens Juice (see p. 153). If you are not consuming these foods, a supplement can effectively provide your body with chlorophyll.

You can buy chlorophyll in liquid or capsule form. I prefer the liquid because when we drink it in water or smoothies, it's penetrating immediately into the body, bypassing the digestive tract. A supplement in pill form can take longer to hit the system and do its work.

Perhaps surprisingly, chlorophyll does not have any taste; however, it turns water a vibrant green color and will stain your tongue—and your clothes, if you spill it. Because of its dark-green tint, I use chlorophyll as a food dye, as do many other natural-food chefs. It's a nontoxic colorant for things like green frosting on a dessert.

Drinking chlorophyll water is something I have committed to doing daily for the rest of my life—and I've done so for more than 10 years. I find this the easiest way to consume it. When I drink chlorophyll water, I like to imagine that I am putting a coating over my cells to protect them from oxidative stress and toxins. Sometimes I visualize myself as a superhero and chlorophyll as my cape. I tell my coaching clients that if they regularly drink alcohol or eat unhealthy food, they should have a chlorophyll water after to help detox the body. Simply add the number of drops recommended on the label to a full glass of water, and drink up!

Copper, Colloidal

Copper is a micronutrient that helps regulate dopamine synthesis and is an essential cofactor for oxidation-reduction reactions in the body. One study found that low copper intake is associated with higher levels of depression and anxiety symptoms.[43] It is naturally occurring in produce like leafy greens (kale, spinach, turnip greens, Swiss chard, and mustard greens), as well as in asparagus, summer squash, legumes, whole grains, nuts, seeds, and seafood.

When taking copper in colloidal supplements—where tiny flecks of copper are suspended in a gel or liquid—be cautious of not consuming too much. You only need a little. Even exceptionally low levels of copper supplementation have been associated with a reduction of symptoms. Follow serving guidelines on the product packaging, and also check with your doctor or other health-care provider because you don't want to take too much. Copper toxicity is in fact linked to a whole host of psychiatric symptoms.

Curcumin, see Turmeric

Essential Oils

Many essential oils can promote reduction of stress and anxiety through aromatherapy. The olfactory sense is directly keyed to the limbic system in the brain, which is associated with the fight-or-flight response and its opposite, the relaxation response. They can be distilled or cold-pressed from specific parts of various plants, such as leaves, peels, petals, or roots, among other things.

The therapeutic properties of scent have been relied upon by folk healers for millennia. I find it fascinating that even the Bible describes Jesus as an infant being visited by three wise men bearing gifts of gold, frankincense, and myrrh! Frankincense and myrrh are tree resins that are often burned as an incense. Having fresh flowers in the home or potted herbs, like lavender or rosemary, can also be a natural way to enjoy the calming benefits of aromatic plants.

You can also use a diffuser to get a beautiful scent of a calming or uplifting essential oil wafting through your home or add essential oils to a nice, relaxing bath. I have a collection of essential oils in my home, which I use to unwind. They always come in handy. I sniff directly from the bottles of oil I keep on my bedside table as needed.

Some essential oils are edible while others are not. For food-grade oils, look for "food-grade" or "therapeutic-grade" on the label. You need to be sure that those you take internally are food-grade and that you trust the purity of the brand before adding them to beverages, like tea or plain water, and to desserts like Genius Chocolate Balls (see p. 246). They can also be combined with an unscented carrier oil, like almond oil, coconut oil, or jojoba oil, or with a lotion and massaged into your skin. (Do not apply straight essential oil to your skin; they must always be diluted in a carrier oil first.)

To reduce tension and anxiety and uplift your spirits, try any or all of these essential oils for aromatherapy:

- Bergamot: Uplifting

- Chamomile: Relaxing

- Clary sage: Sedative

- Copaiba: Comforting (Like CBD oil, copaiba binds with the brain's cannabidiol receptors. It contains no THC and does not get you "high.")

- Frankincense: Sedative

- Geranium: Calming

- Jasmine: Emotionally healing

- Lavender: Calming

- Lemon: Uplifting

- Lemon balm, aka Melissa: Sedative

- Myrrh: Relaxing

- Neroli: Soothing

- Orange: Uplifting

- Patchouli: Sedative

- Petitgrain: Calming (It has chemical properties similar to lavender with the floral scent.)

- Rose: Soothing

- Valerian: Relaxing

- Ylang-ylang: Sedative

FISH OIL, SEE OMEGA-3 FATTY ACIDS

FOLATE, SEE B-COMPLEX VITAMINS

GABA (GAMMA-AMINOBUTYRIC ACID)

See pages 20 to 21 for information about GABA and how to increase your levels of this important calming neurotransmitter.

GOLD, COLLOIDAL

Gold taken internally is healing! Yes, the same gold we wear in jewelry is able to be ingested in specific quantities (nanoparticles). Recently, gold has been actively used in different spheres for diagnostic and therapeutic purposes.[44] Studies have been devoted to the interaction between the cells of the immune system and gold nanoparticles.[45]

A relatively new supplement on the market, colloidal gold is said to be helpful in treating depression, anxiety, and addiction, reducing inflammation, and improving gut health. Taking colloidal gold internally has been done as far back as the 4th and 5th centuries B.C.E. when the first mentions are found in treatises by Chinese, Arabian, and Indian scientists. In Europe during the Middle Ages, colloidal gold was studied and used in alchemist laboratories. Paracelsus, a 16th-century Swiss physician, wrote about the therapeutic properties of gold quintessence, and he used it in the treatment of a number of mental diseases.[46]

Where gold comes into the anxiety picture is in its capacity for relieving stress, repairing the brain, and boosting the immune response of the body to oxidative stress. Europeans have long used colloidal gold as a supplement in the diet, but modern usage of colloidal gold supplements is generally for joint health. Some contemporary researchers have concluded that colloidal gold has an incredibly positive effect on nerve structure and the brain![47]

HOLY BASIL (TULSI)

Holy basil, or tulsi, is an aromatic perennial plant native to India that is used by herbalists to treat stress, anxiety, fatigue, headaches, and inflammation. It has anti-inflammatory and anti-oxidant properties as well as immunomodulatory effects—meaning, it produces antibodies.[48] One study has shown that it boosts cognition and reduces anxiety traits.[49] Holy basil is an adaptogen that can assist us in coping with stress. The findings from 24 human studies suggest that holy basil is a safe herbal intervention for psychological and immunological stress.[50]

Holy basil normalizes neurotransmitter levels in the brain. A 2009 study in India demonstrated a 39 percent reduction of symptoms of stress (insomnia, heart palpitations, headaches, fatigue, irritability, sexual dysfunction, gastrointestinal distress, and more) over a six-week period with participants taking 1,200 milligrams per day of holy basil.[51]

You can enjoy a relaxing cup of tea made with the leaves of holy basil or use a powdered herbal supplement.

INOSITOL, SEE B-COMPLEX VITAMINS

KAVA KAVA (*PIPER METHYSTICUM*)

Kava kava (kava for short) contains kavapyrones, substances that act much like alcohol on your brain, making you feel calm, relaxed, and happy. The plant is also thought to relieve pain, prevent seizures, and relax muscles. A drink made from kava root has been consumed in many cultures for centuries because it is known to relieve anxiety, restlessness, and insomnia.[52] Several studies have demonstrated that kava is an anxiolytic agent.[53]

The first randomized, placebo-controlled, double-blind study of kava for the treatment of patients who were diagnosed with anxiety disorder was conducted in 1997. The subjects were given either an extract of kava or a placebo for 25 weeks. Those who were given the kava extract showed improvement in their primary and secondary anxiety symptoms. Primary symptoms observed were nervousness, restlessness, and fatigue. Secondary symptoms included sweating, rapid heartbeat, and having a sense of impending danger. Besides verifying its general effectiveness in relieving anxiety, the researchers also concluded that when kava was used as an alternative to pharmaceutical medications like benzodiazepines and tricyclic antidepressants, individuals typically suffered from fewer unwanted side effects.[54]

You can buy kava as an herbal supplement online and in health food stores. Sometimes it is blended with other ingredients in products labeled as stress response supplements.

Caution: Don't take kava kava and operate heavy machinery.

Lemon Balm (*Melissa officinalis*)

Lemon balm is a lemon-scented herb in the mint family. It has traditionally been used to improve mood and cognitive function and as a sleep aid and digestive tonic. It promotes calmness and reduces stress and anxiety.

Records concerning the medicinal use of lemon balm date back more than 2,000 years. Renaissance Swiss physician Paracelsus (1493 to 1541 c.e.), an early chemist who has been called the father of toxicology, noted that lemon balm could completely "revivify" a man and recommended it be used for "all complaints supposed to proceed from a disordered state of the nervous system."[55]

Lemon balm is available in tea, herbal extract, and essential oil form. These can be added to water, coffee, shakes, smoothies, or salad dressings. If you're feeling jittery, try applying lemon balm/melissa in a lotion to your skin, which feels lovely and soothing. You also could take an Epsom salt (magnesium) bath with a few drops of essential oil added, and then, for good measure, put lemon balm lotion on your skin afterward and climb into bed.

Tip: You could grow your own lemon balm at home! It is easy to grow at home in a pot or in your garden, as long as it gets direct sunlight. Not only do its leaves have a rich, zippy lemon scent, but lemon balm also contains compounds that can repel mosquitoes. For a quick homemade mosquito repellent, simply crush a handful of lemon balm leaves in your hand and rub them on your exposed skin. Fewer mosquitos, less anxiety? It's worth a try!

LICORICE ROOT

The history of licorice root can be dated to 2300 B.C.E. Folk healers thought licorice to be a magic plant that rejuvenated aging people. A sweet flavor can be extracted from the licorice root, one that we may know from the licorice candy or alcoholic beverages like ouzo, which comes from Greece. Licorice root contains glycyrrhizic acid, which causes it to be anti-inflammatory and immune boosting. It is classed as an adaptogen—it helps us cope with stress. It is also used to soothe gastrointestinal problems. The results obtained in one study of its emotional impact support the hypothesis that licorice eases anxiety.[56]

A group of researchers at Pusan National University in Korea investigated the effect of licorice on the memory and cognition of rodents with inflammation, as they were curious about the role of inflammation in neurodegenerative disorders, such as anxiety. Their results showed licorice as a favorable therapeutic agent.[57] Since we believe inflammation contributes to anxiety, it makes sense we should consider supplementation with licorice extract for anxiety.

I'm obviously not talking about licorice candy, so don't go eating a ton of black licorice thinking it will reduce anxiety, as the sugar and preservatives in candy will do the reverse.

You can take licorice in supplement form, as a liquid extract, or as tea.

Caution: Ask your doctor before taking licorice in large amounts. Long-term use can cause high blood pressure and low potassium levels, which could lead to heart and muscle problems. Licorice may also interfere with some medications.

LYSINE, SEE AMINO ACIDS

MAGNESIUM

Magnesium is a naturally occurring mineral found in food that's known to relax the brain and body. It is beneficial in the treatment of migraines, insomnia, anxiety, depression, and coronary artery disease.[58] Yet experts say that up to 75 percent of people in United States are not meeting their recommended intake of magnesium![59] Could this be a contributing factor in why so many are suffering with anxiety? Yes, magnesium deficiency has been shown to cause anxiety.[60] One study found 75 percent of depressed patients to be magnesium deficient, with another 9 percent at borderline levels.[61]

Supplementation with magnesium has been shown to directly reduce stress and anxiety. An efficacy trial showed that magnesium supplements may be a fast, safe, and easily accessible alternative, or adjunct, to starting or increasing the dose of antidepressant medications.[62]

You should regularly consume magnesium-rich foods, and the recipes in this book provide guidance on how to build recipes from ingredients that do this. But I would also recommend taking a magnesium supplement. Magnesium is one of my personal favorite antianxiety supplements. After I started taking them, the feelings of depression and anxiety I was experiencing were reduced and my sleep improved.

The main reason people are deficient in magnesium is due to low dietary intake. Check with your doctor if you are deficient, and then you can supplement if you are. Follow the labels on the back of magnesium supplement bottles for recommended dosages. Intravenous magnesium is also available to people who are extremely deficient.

Fun fact: You can take a magnesium bath! Simply add Epsom salt (magnesium sulfate) to your bathwater or a footbath. The magnesium can be absorbed through your skin while also relaxing your muscles and relieving tension.

I recommend taking Epsom salt baths once a week to relieve some anxiety. Add ½ cup to 2 cups of Epsom salt that has been drizzled with essential oils (try lavender) to a warm or hot bath. Soak for 10 to 20 minutes. I do this often, and it really helps me wind down. (Let someone know you are going in the bath beforehand as it may cause lightheadedness.)

MELATONIN

Melatonin is a hormone primarily released by the pineal gland. It regulates the sleep-wake cycle, improving sleep quality, regulating circadian rhythm, and easing negative feelings associated with anxiousness. It is primarily released by the pineal gland. Melatonin is also a potent antioxidant and free radical scavenger.[63]

As a supplement, melatonin is often used for the short-term treatment of trouble sleeping, such as from jet lag or shift work. It is known for helping people feel calm at bedtime, so they get better sleep. The National Sleep Foundation recommends a dosage of between 0.2 and 5 milligrams for adults each day, which is best to take one hour before going to bed.[64]

Melatonin has been in many human trials and studies, and some researchers say it is appropriate to offer instead of benzodiazepines (familiar names for this type of medication include Valium and Xanax). Melatonin was proved equally as effective as the standard treatment with midazolam (sedative) in reducing preoperative anxiety in adults![65]

Naturally occurring melatonin has been reported in fruits and vegetables, including tart cherries, corn, asparagus, bananas, tomatoes, pomegranate, olives, broccoli, cucumbers, grapes, and plums; grains such as rice, barley, and oats; walnuts and peanuts; sunflower seeds, mustard seeds, and flaxseed; as well as in herbs, olive oil, wine, and beer. When we consume foods rich in melatonin, such as banana, pineapple, and orange, our blood levels of melatonin increase significantly.

For a while in the early 2000s, melatonin-infused beverages and snacks were being sold in grocery stores, convenience stores, and even clubs![66] However, the Food and Drug Administration cracked down on many of the makers; although melatonin was a legal supplement, it was not approved as a food additive.[67] Today, you can take melatonin supplements, liquid melatonin, or a spray under your tongue.

Caution: Taking too much melatonin is said to lead to grogginess the next day. It can also make some drugs less effective, including high blood pressure medications and, potentially, birth control pills.[68]

Niacin (Vitamin B₃), see B-Complex Vitamins

Omega-3 Fatty Acids

Omega-3 fats are the fats the brain thrives on. Research has shown that people who consume more omega-3s from foods or supplements may have a lower risk of developing anxiety, depression, and other problems with cognitive function.[69]

There are three main omega-3 fatty acids:

- Alpha-linolenic acid (ALA): Found mainly in plant oils such as flaxseed, soybean, and canola oils.

- Eicosapentaenoic acid (EPA): Found mainly in fish.

- Docosahexaenoic acid (DHA): Found mainly in fish.

Supplementation with omega-3 fatty acids is a practical way to increase their levels in your body, especially for those who do not eat fish. Omega-3 dietary supplements usually include fish oil, krill oil, and cod liver oil, all of which come in a wide range of doses. If you're a vegan or prefer a vegetarian option, you can get your supplemental omega-3s from flaxseed oil, hemp oil, marine algae oil, spirulina, or chlorella.

Fish oil was the first supplement my doctor recommended to me when my blood test showed I had low omega-3 levels. This supplement alone can help reduce anxiety fairly effectively.

Experts have not established recommended amounts for omega-3s except for ALA. The amount you need depends on your age and sex. Children need between 0.5 grams and 1.6 grams of ALA daily. Adults need between 1.1 and 1.6 grams daily.

PASSIONFLOWER

Passionflower has a long history of use as an anxiolytic agent in folklore and has been used by people all over the world.[70] In the 1970s through the 1990s, passionflower was listed as an official plant drug by the pharmacopoeias of America, Britain, Germany, France, Switzerland, Egypt, and India; its wide use has made it an acceptable treatment for restlessness and nervousness.[71]

To date, three human trials have documented the efficacy of passionflower as a treatment for anxiety-related disorders.[72] One double-blind, placebo-controlled study analyzed the difference in efficacy between oxazepam (a prescription benzodiazepine used to treat chronic anxiety symptoms) and passionflower in patients who met the criteria for an anxiety disorder.[73] The results showed no difference between the two anxiolytics with regard to the treatment of anxiety, suggesting that passionflower is as effective as benzodiazepines in eliminating anxiety symptoms! Subjects from the passionflower group also reported lower job performance impairment than those in the benzodiazepine group; however, subjects in the benzodiazepine group reported a faster onset of symptom relief.

You can get passionflower herbal supplements, liquid extract, or tea.

PREBIOTICS

Prebiotics are food ingredients that encourage the growth and activity of beneficial microorganisms (see "Probiotics") so we can establish a healthy microbiome in our digestive tracts. *Biotic* means "related to living things." Prebiotic compounds are what probiotic microbes themselves like to eat—typically, nondigestible fiber. You can get prebiotics naturally from tigernuts, asparagus, bananas, and garlic or you can buy commercially prepared prebiotics in powder or capsule forms. They are another supplement to support good gut health so our brain can be healthier.

PROBIOTICS

Pro means "for." *Bio* means "life." The aptly named probiotics promote life.

Probiotics are the good bacteria in the human gut that help us get our vitamins and microorganisms. You get them naturally when you eat fermented foods, kombucha, miso, tempeh, sourdough, and raw milk and raw or fermented milk products. At present, it is commonly accepted that probiotic products are generally safe and can improve health, although the immunocompromised, elderly, and chronically ill should seek guidance from their doctor.[74]

Imbalance of gut microbes has been implicated in many disorders—everything from inflammatory bowel disease to obesity, psychiatric illnesses (including anxiety), and different cancers. As a supplement that helps the gut function properly, probiotics play a role in protecting us against gut-brain–connected anxiety.

Gut health is paramount to optimal wellness, and I believe that probiotics are something we all should explore for achieving that. If you try probiotics for a month and feel better, then you'll have your answer as to whether they work for you. I felt better almost immediately after starting to take probiotics, so I know they work very well for me personally.

For a good supplement, I recommend buying the ones that come in the refrigerated section of the store, and then keeping them in your fridge at home. This is because probiotic bacteria are naturally sensitive to heat and moisture. Heat can kill microorganisms. If I am traveling, then I take probiotics with me that don't need to be refrigerated because I would rather have those than none at all.

RHODIOLA

Rhodiola rosea is a perennial flowering plant that is used as a supplement for increasing energy, stamina, strength, and mental capacity, and as an adaptogen to help the body cope with and resist physical, chemical, and environmental stress, thus helping to reduce anxiety.

Historically, people have used rhodiola for anxiety, fatigue, anemia, impotence, infections, headache, and depression related to stress. People also have used it to increase physical endurance, work performance, and longevity, and to improve resistance to high-altitude sickness. Today people use rhodiola as a dietary supplement to increase energy, stamina, and strength, to improve attention and memory, and to enhance the ability to cope with stress.[75]

A trial was done to evaluate the impact of a *Rhodiola rosea* L. extract on self-reported anxiety, stress, cognition, and other mood symptoms of 80 mildly anxious participants who were given a 200-milligram dose of rhodiola twice a day—once before breakfast and once before lunch—for two weeks. At the end of the study, participants reported having significant reductions in anxiety, stress, anger, confusion, depression, and overall mood. It's amazing what can change for us in only 14 days![76]

You can take rhodiola supplements, liquid extract, and tea. You can also add it to your smoothies. It's best to take rhodiola on an empty stomach, but not before bed, as it has a slight stimulatory effect. Follow the instructions on the product package for appropriate dosage.

Caution: Check with your doctor before taking rhodiola, and do not take it if you are pregnant or nursing or taking prescription monoamine oxidase inhibitors (MAOIs).

SCHISANDRA, OR SCHIZANDRA (*SCHISANDRA CHINENSIS*)

Schisandra is a woody vine that bears vibrant red fruits called magnolia berries. The purple-red berries are described as having five tastes: sweet, salty, bitter, pungent, and sour. The berry is used to make an adaptogenic medicine that increases one's resistance to disease and stress symptoms while increasing energy and physical endurance.[77] It counters stress by reducing the levels of stress hormones, such as cortisol, in the blood.[78]

You can take schisandra tablets, liquid extract, or tea. Follow the recommended dosage on the package. Dried schisandra berries also can be purchased online and eaten like dried goji berries as a snack, or added to smoothies, desserts, açai bowls, and cereal. Schisandra powder, berries, and seeds are often used to make tonics and teas. You can add any of these to your smoothies.

Tip: Try using schisandra tea as an unconventional, but highly effective, coffee alternative for an early morning jump-start or as a caffeine-free energy boost in the afternoon.

Silver, Colloidal

Colloidal silver is a liquid or gel in which microscopic particles of silver are suspended.[79] Silver is naturally found in soil, mushrooms, and breast milk. And yes, it's the same metal we wear as jewelry. As a dietary supplement, silver can be safely consumed in small quantities in colloidal form. The liquid contains only nanoparticles of the metal.

Poor-quality preparations of colloidal silver and over-consumption of the product can cause a condition known as *argyria*, which causes the skin to turn ashy blue. Good-quality colloidal silver preparations taken in appropriately small doses do not turn the skin blue. *Do not make your own at home.* Avoid impure products with additives and adhere strictly to the packaging guidelines.[80]

Robert Scott Bell, host of his eponymous radio show and co-author of *Unlock the Power to Heal*, says: "Colloidal silver repairs the skin faster than anything else on the planet. There is nothing on earth that causes skin regrowth like colloidal silver, and second place is aloe, and that's why the combination is so great for healing the gut or any wounds. Silver is the great accelerator in tissue regeneration. It works by taking damaged cells out of a damaged state and replacing them with healthy new cells. And that is why silver is a mainstay in burn centers around the world."[81] Colloidal silver has been used for centuries by natural healers to treat infections due to yeast, bacteria, parasites, and viruses. Modern research studies are beginning to assess colloidal silver with positive results.[82]

The reason colloidal silver is helpful with anxiety is that it helps to boost the immune system and assists with good gut health. As was discussed earlier, people with compromised immune systems often experience anxiety, so taking supplements to strengthen immunity are most beneficial.

You can spray colloidal silver under your tongue for 30 seconds three times a day or put the liquid under your tongue where it is swiftly absorbed. You could also do the Aloe and Colloidal Silver Protocol (see p. 69).

Spirulina, see Blue-Green Algae

St. John's Wort

St. John's wort is an herbal remedy derived from the flowering tops of a perennial shrub and has been used in traditional folk medicine for centuries to treat a wide range of disorders. In Germany, it is accepted as a complementary treatment for anxiety, depression, and sleep disorders.[83]

Many studies suggest that St. John's wort is effective in alleviating mild to moderate depression. The Mayo Clinic says "some research has shown the supplement to be as effective as several prescription antidepressants."[84] A study of 149 patients with depression with both anxiety and obsessive-compulsive disorder (OCD) demonstrated that six weeks of treatment with St. John's wort significantly reduced anxiety.[85]

You can take St. John's wort supplements, liquid extract, and tea.

Caution: St. John's wort is well known for having serious interactions with a wide variety of medications, including antidepressants.[86] Do not take this supplement without first consulting with your doctor.

THEANINE, SEE AMINO ACIDS

THIAMINE, SEE B-COMPLEX VITAMINS

TRYPTOPHAN, SEE AMINO ACIDS

TULSI, SEE HOLY BASIL

TURMERIC

Turmeric and its active component, curcumin, have been well studied for their neuroprotective and anti-inflammatory effects. Curcumin modulates various neurotransmitter levels in the brain and has anxiolytic effects on biochemical and behavioral symptoms associated with anxiety. (For a more thorough discussion of the health benefits of turmeric and its main active component, curcumin, see Chapter 2.)

Rather than eating turmeric, some people prefer to take turmeric supplements so they can ensure they are consuming it every day. It's important to note that turmeric powder contains only about 3 percent curcumin. For this reason, many people choose to take curcumin supplements, rather than turmeric, to harness more of its antioxidant and anti-inflammatory effects.

Follow the recommend serving on the back of any turmeric or curcumin supplements that you get.

Tyrosine, see Amino Acids

Zinc

Zinc deficiency can cause anxiety. The most substantial amounts of zinc are found in the part of our brain that controls mood. Zinc is needed to create neurotransmitters. Studies demonstrate that zinc therapy is effective in increasing zinc plasma levels and that zinc supplementation may play a role in improving symptoms associated with anxiety.[87] Results have reportedly found zinc deficiency in patients with depression and anxiety and have suggested zinc for therapy to improve mental health. You can check with your doctor to see if you have a zinc deficiency, and if so, you can consider supplementation.

Alternatively, eat foods high in zinc, such as shellfish, meat, legumes like chickpeas, beans and lentils, seeds, nuts, eggs, whole grains, and dairy.

Liana's Top Six Antianxiety Supplements

These are my favorite supplements! I personally use them every day.

1. Chlorophyll

2. Fish oil

3. Spirulina

4. Gold, colloidal

5. Magnesium

6. St. John's wort

I continue to discover more information about important supplements every day! To learn about supplements such as 5-HTP, echinacea, bilberry, gingko biloba, and more, please go to my website, www.LianaWernerGray.com/AnxietyFree, where I'll share all the latest research with you. You can also read about the Anxiety-Free supplements that I developed at LianaWernergray.com/AnxietyFreeSupps.

CHAPTER 4

The Most Neurotoxic Foods on the Planet

The quality and composition of the food we eat are under constant scrutiny, and so they should be. It is appalling that we see certain so-called food being sold. I say "so-called" because this type of food is not genuinely nourishing. The foods I discuss in this chapter are those you should attempt to phase out of your diet altogether.

In general, a processed-food lifestyle is not one that will sustain you for a lifetime. It harms the brain—it's *neurotoxic*—and has been proven to cause anxiety and other health problems. So many of us have gotten used to this way of eating; it often seems easier, more convenient, cheaper, exciting, and, yes, even tasty. But if you eat this way for the long term, your mind and body will suffer. Constantly eating processed foods leads to constant anxiety.

To call some of the following foods "food" seems disrespectful to real ingredients that come from the plant and animal kingdoms, as many are created in a lab and are poisonous. These Frankenfoods are created with extreme levels of processing or in a laboratory, using synthesized chemicals. In a nutshell, they are lacking a wholesome chemical structure that is harmonious with the systems nature devised for our bodies. As a consequence, these foods cause anxiety and negative mood swings.

To make it easy for you to remember what to avoid, just know that if a food has been far removed from nature, or wasn't even derived from nature at all, it is not good for you. It places a burden on the body. Science has proven these things cause anxiety and worse: cancer and depression—even suicidal thoughts.

This is a serious chapter, but it warrants reading because food should be a serious part of our health-care strategy.

Baby Steps on the Path to Health

Some people may look at the list in this chapter and say it is too "extreme" to cut out their (current) favorite foods from their diets. My favorite part about the work I do is helping people find nutritional solutions that enable them to enjoy eating healthy foods more frequently—or every day—and reaping incredible benefits to mind, body, and spirit! That's why in the very next chapter, I offer simple solutions for improving choices in every food group we most enjoy. Would you be willing to take a transitional step of upgrading your choices, rather than just cutting these things out completely right away? You can continue to enjoy delicious meals and snacks without eating Frankenfood, so please understand that I am not advocating a gloom-and-doom scenario.

Remember as well that you're reading this book because you or someone you love experiences anxiety, irritability, mood swings, depression, and low energy, and possibly brain fog, confusion, or lack of ability to concentrate. Cutting these foods out of your diet doesn't have to make you miserable. In fact, just the opposite is true. You will feel so much better once your body detoxes from them and begins to receive proper nourishment. Yes, avoiding neurotoxic foods may require that you make a drastic lifestyle change, but that is the end goal. Sometimes it's easiest to make a gradual transition. But do keep your mind and intentions on the end goal as you learn how to eat better.

The "Why" Behind Neurotoxic Foods

There are several reasons the foods I highlight in this chapter are the worst for anxiety:

- They are anxiogenic, which means they are anxiety producing. Researchers have measured the anxiogenic effects of many different foods and ingredients.

- They cause oxidative stress and inflammation. The brain is especially vulnerable to free radicals because its functions are more oriented to fats than antioxidant resources.[1]

- They are endocrine disruptors. The endocrine system is the system of glands that produce hormones, which regulate mood and sleep, among other things. Disrupting the endocrine system creates hormonal imbalances that contribute to anxiety.

- They weaken the immune system. In this state, our energy is low and our susceptibility to infectious diseases is raised. Emotionally, being unwell is unsettling.

- They are neurotoxic, which means they are destructive to brain cells and nerves.

Neurotoxins affect function in both developing and mature brains and bodies and include both human-made and natural substances—everything from pesticides and industrial solvents to ethanol (drinking alcohol), botulinum toxin (Botox), lead, mercury, and manganese. Food poisoning can result from biological compounds such as tetrodotoxin and domoic acid from contaminated mussels and other shellfish, or monosodium glutamate, a common additive to bump up flavor in snack foods. Overexposure to neurotoxins causes neurotoxicity, which can lead to damage of the brain and peripheral nervous system, including disruption of nerve function or nerve death.

Symptoms of neurotoxicity include cognitive and behavioral problems: headaches; limb weakness or numbness; loss of memory, vision, and/or intellect; uncontrollable obsessive and/or compulsive behaviors; sexual dysfunction; delusions; anxiety; and depression. Medical treatment involves eliminating or reducing exposure to the toxic substance once it is identified. A diet of clean food without pesticides and additives, in my opinion, should be part of treatment.

So many people think they are "crazy" when they experience anxiety, depression, and mood disorders, but I believe some may be experiencing symptoms of toxicity. The environments we live in and the foods we eat are major contributors to our mental and emotional health that we should factor in when creating our treatment plans.

If you think you have neurotoxicity, ask your doctor to get tests done. It is said the best kind of test is one that shows whether the peripheral nervous system has been affected. Tests to detect damage to the brain may include pupillography (the study of pupils in the eyes), heart-rate-variability stress testing, brain imaging with the triple-camera SPECT system, and neuropsychological testing.[2]

Recovery from neurotoxicity depends upon the length and degree of exposure and the severity of the neurological injury. In some instances, exposure can be fatal. In others, patients may survive yet not fully recover. In other situations, individuals recover completely. Best not to roll the dice in the first place, and instead to be kind to our brains and bodies. It is crucial to be careful with your diet and to eat the foods that restore and sustain your cognitive and nervous system function. Neurotoxins are all around us, but they are especially common in popular processed and prepared foods.

It's important to remember, however, that it's not the end of the world to occasionally consume the toxic foods described in this chapter. As the saying goes, it's the dose that makes the poison. One study on food toxins put it this way: "Historically, we have learned that everything is toxic; it is only the dose that separates the toxic from the non-toxic. Even water is toxic if a large amount (four to five liters) is consumed in a relatively short time (two to three hours)."[3] In other words, at normal levels of consumption, there is little potential for toxicity from natural food toxins. So if you slip up, it's okay! You can make better choices with your next meal. If you can't eliminate a food entirely, it's okay! Just do what you can to the best of your ability and with the resources that you have. (And be sure to read Chapter 5 very carefully to fully absorb the food upgrade mindset!)

Top 6 "Controversial" Foods

In my research, I came across some conflicting arguments on a few foods, which I'm going to call controversial, or suspicious, foods. It's a head-scratcher. There are researchers and doctors who say they reduce anxiety, while others suggest they increase anxiety. (Some of these foods were even discussed in previous chapters!) Let's talk about these to start, before getting into the definitely horrible foods.

Suspect #1. Aged, Fermented, Cured, Smoked, and Cultured Foods: Cheese, Kefir, Kimchi, Pickles, Salami, Sauerkraut, Red Wine, Soy Sauce, and Yogurt

Some experts say that aged, fermented, and cultured foods cause anxiety; however, foods of this type have also been proven healthy for the gut—thus possibly helping to reduce anxiety and depression. Here's what we know.

It is said that in the process of fermentation, bacteria break down food protein into biogenic amines, one of which is histamine. Histamine is a neurotransmitter that is involved with processes of digestion, hormones, and the cardiovascular and nervous systems. It is part of the body's natural defense against invaders. Sometimes too much is released, which triggers inflammation and anxiety.

Even though Suspect #1–type foods bolster biogenic amines, a study published in the journal *Psychiatry Research* found a link between probiotic foods and a lowering of social anxiety.[4] Another study linked probiotics with improving symptoms of major depressive disorder, saying they do this by decreasing inflammation in the body and/or by increasing the availability of the calming brain chemical serotonin.[5]

Bottom line: I believe these foods are safe when consumed in moderation if your digestive system is currently in balance. Their safety depends on each person's gut health. Personally, I believe that probiotic foods have been a positive factor in my gut and mental health. While supplements can provide probiotics, it's nice to know they can also be sourced through whole foods.

Suspect #2. Alcohol: Liquor, Beer, and Wine

It is believed that drinking any kind of alcohol in excess can cause anxiety, whereas drinking alcohol in moderation, most particularly wine, may reduce stress and ease anxiety.

A study of the Mediterranean diet showed that moderate consumption of wine reduced the incidence of depression.[6] One review suggested that "alcohol in moderate amounts is effective in reducing stress [by] both physiologic and self-report measures." The researchers also described low and moderate doses of alcohol as increasing "pleasant and carefree feelings" while decreasing "tension, depression, and self-consciousness." I was fascinated to read that heavy drinkers and also *abstainers* may have higher rates of clinical depression than do regular moderate drinkers.[7]

Another recent study, however, had very concerning results. The researchers focused on adults over the age of 50 with a "Mediterranean drinking pattern" of moderate alcohol intake and a preference for wine. They suggested there were inconsistencies in the literature and concluded: "Our results do not support the presence of a protective effect derived from moderate alcohol consumption in general, and wine in particular, on the risk of developing depression or psychological distress among older adults."[8]

Psychotherapist Mike Dow, Psy.D., Ph.D., says that one alcoholic drink per day (two for men) may help keep toxins out of the brain, reducing a person's risk of dementia by as much as 23 percent! The benefits hold for all types of alcohol, but studies show wine, particularly red wine, works best. On his website, Dr. Dow writes, "The red grape skin is rich in a potent antioxidant called resveratrol, and among red wines, pinot noir has very high levels. If you prefer a lighter drink, try champagne. Research suggests the phenolic acid it contains may prove a powerful weapon to help you think better. A glass of red wine with dinner may lessen blood-sugar spikes by preventing intestinal glucose absorption and reducing your liver's production of glucose."[9]

People always ask me what the healthiest alcohol is to drink, and the easiest way to know is to ask, "How is it processed?" Remember, minimally processed ingredients that are close to their natural state are usually the healthiest. A wine that comes from the grape is great and proven to have health benefits, tequila comes from the agave cactus, and you can get a good vodka from potatoes.

Bottom line: Finding your unique balance is important. What is not too much, and perhaps not too little, alcohol for your unique body? Where is the ideal middle ground? Too much alcohol too much of the time can't be good.

Suspect #3. Caffeine: Coffee, Nonherbal Tea, Cacao, and Chocolate

Caffeine is the most widely consumed psychoactive drug in the world. Natural sources of caffeine include coffee, tea, and chocolate. Cacao, which has small amounts of caffeine in it, has been proven to be powerful in reducing anxiety and depression. Data obtained from human clinical trials indicated that coffee exhibits protective effects against brain diseases, including Alzheimer's disease, Parkinson's disease, and amyotrophic lateral sclerosis (ALS).[10]

Some say caffeine is an enemy and causes anxiety; however, there also have been studies showing that coffee is neuroprotective and has health benefits in regard to anxiety. When determining whether caffeine is right for you, keep in mind the study published in *Psychiatry Research*, which shows that people with anxiety disorder tend to have increased caffeine sensitivity.[11]

Caffeine isn't good for all body types. A study reported that for healthy adults, caffeine consumption is relatively safe, but that for some it could contribute to impairments in cardiovascular function, sleep, and substance use.[12] Some people's bodies just don't tolerate it well. Also, if you have been under constant stress for a while and have adrenal fatigue, it's not a good idea to consume caffeine. Too much caffeine can deplete neurotransmitters and burn out the adrenal glands, which are associated with the fight-or-flight response.

Another study I've read suggests that secondary students are adversely affected by high doses of caffeine, so I believe coffee should be restricted to adults.[13] Pregnant women and younger children may also be vulnerable to the negative effects of caffeine.

Bottom line: I personally enjoy a bit of caffeine every day, usually from cacao. I will also enjoy caffeine in green tea and black tea. I believe that caffeine is not the enemy. It's only troublesome if we have too much of it.

If you do choose to enjoy coffee, keep it to no more than once a day. If you feel like you have had too much caffeine, consider abstaining for a month to give your body a break and then reassess how you feel when you ingest it. Personally, I believe that coffee is one of nature's best gifts and can assist us in living a healthy, energized, and joyful life when used in balance.

Suspect #4. Dairy: Milk, Cream, Butter, Cheese, Kefir, and Yogurt

In my research, I found some experts who say dairy—including fermented kinds of dairy (kefir and yogurt)—causes anxiety. Other experts say that some dairy helps to relieve stress, a factor we want to keep low as it can sometimes trigger anxiety. Do the benefits outweigh the costs? Here's what we know.

Dairy contains important nutrients. It is a source of calcium, vitamin D, protein, phosphorus, and a host of micronutrients that are said to promote skeletal, muscular, and neurologic development.[14] Dairy has also been linked to relaxation. One study shows that consuming dairy reduces anger and is associated with positive mental health.[15] Another study shows that increased dairy consumption attenuates both oxidative and inflammatory stress.[16]

But dairy also has inflammatory properties. For some people, casein—a protein found in dairy products—is the problem. It triggers inflammation in the brain.[17] It also has been known to wreak havoc on the digestive system, causing bloating, diarrhea, constipation, IBS, and leaky gut. Dr. Dow says that dairy is inflammatory and can contribute to brain fog.[18] Psychiatrist Kelly Brogan believes that dairy sabotages the brain.[19]

Other research shows that people who have anxiety say they've noticed an increase in anxiety symptoms within mere minutes of consuming dairy products. In one study, episodic movement disorders (that is, shaking the head from side to side) were reported after the consumption of skim milk. This adverse reaction was attributed to the high content of L-tyrosine in dairy products.[20]

Bottom line: I believe the benefits of dairy, particularly raw and raw fermented products, outweigh the downsides for some people. Personally, I do not take dairy well. My body doesn't feel good when I eat it, and my mood feels more "down." I eat dairy once every two months or so, usually in the form of organic cheese on a pizza. This is a good balance for me. By contrast, I know people who feel so comforted and delighted when consuming dairy. You must find that balance for you.

If you suspect dairy is causing gut issues or anxiety for you, I recommend doing a 30-day elimination and then reassessing how you feel afterward.

Suspect #5. Gluten: Wheat, Barley, and Rye

Gluten is a protein naturally found in wheat, barley, and rye. It acts as a binder, holding food together and adding a "stretchy" quality to it. The most wholesome and healthy way to consume gluten is in a nice piece of organic bread.

Problems arise if one has digestive issues like IBS, celiac disease, leaky gut, or dysbiosis. People with celiac disease cannot tolerate gluten because it triggers an immune response that damages the lining of the small intestine. Holly Strawbridge, former executive director of the *Harvard Health Letter*, explains: "This can interfere with the absorption of nutrients from food, cause a host of symptoms, and lead to other problems like osteoporosis, infertility, nerve damage, and seizures."[21] But even people with milder allergies can find the glue-like starch triggering. A meta-analysis that included 3 randomized trials and 10 studies concluded that eliminating gluten was an effective treatment strategy for mood disorders in gluten-sensitive individuals.[22]

Gluten is a suspect in most health issues, as it affects the gut, which also affects the brain. Does it cause anxiety? It's possible. If you have a healthy gut microbiome, consuming gluten may be fine for you as long as it comes from high-quality organic and non-GMO sources. Dr. Mike Dow, however, recommends eliminating gluten, as it can cause brain fog.

Bottom line: I recommend experimenting with cutting gluten from your diet for 30 days, paying attention the entire time to how you feel. Some people I counsel on nutrition report that they feel sharper and less anxious, and have way more energy when they cut gluten from their diets. If you have an imbalance of microflora or yeast in your digestive tract, you shouldn't eat gluten; give your gut at least a 12-month break from it.

Find your own balance, too. I don't recommend eating gluten every day, even if you do have a healthy gut; and I certainly don't recommend eating processed foods like cakes and cookies that contain gluten either. Perhaps look at gluten foods more as treats. I will enjoy some gluten once every two weeks or so, usually by having a slice or two of organic bread. This is the right balance for me. During the period when I was initially healing my anxiety, I didn't eat anything with gluten in it for six months. Now that my health is restored and my gut is functioning optimally, I can take gluten a little more often.

In conclusion, as always, you must find your own balance with gluten. Discovering what works for your body may be a process of trial and error.

Suspect #6. Nightshades: Potatoes, Tomatoes, Eggplant, Peppers, and Goji Berries

There is speculation among some researchers that plants in the nightshade family cause anxiety.[23] Nightshade foods contain trace amounts of solanine, a poisonous compound that some people believe aggravates arthritis pain and inflammation. Nightshade foods are also said to be problematic for people with autoimmune diseases due to their lectin, saponin, and capsaicin content. People who have an intolerance to nightshade plants aren't able to digest them fully. They usually experience gas, bloating, headaches, fatigue, joint pain, and anxiety. However, there is also plenty of evidence for the neuroprotective effects of certain members of the nightshade family, especially tomatoes!

Bottom line: While I do believe that nightshades aren't a good fit for every person, for many of us they are healthy and nutritionally beneficial. If you suspect they may affect you, cut nightshades from your diet for a month and track your mood and health.

* * *

Remember to respect your bioindividuality by tuning in to what your body is trying to tell you. Just as I've asked you to assess how you feel when introducing any new food, assess how you feel when you remove a substance from your life. Check in with yourself to see if your needs change and you can no longer tolerate something you once could, or vice versa. If anything isn't right for your metabolism or current physical condition, you are better off cutting it out of your diet completely. Eat something delicious that makes you feel fantastic instead!

THE MOST NEUROTOXIC FOODS ON THE PLANET

Hippocrates, widely regarded as the father of medicine, once said: "Let your food be your medicine, and your medicine be your food." The following foods are certainly not "medicine"; they are chronic stressors that remodel our brains in negative ways. Although you may not die right away after eating them, they have been proven to deteriorate the brain and other bodily tissues, so I don't believe we want to take their toxicity lightly. They aren't derived from natural food sources, so the moderation and balance rule we used with the controversial foods doesn't apply anymore.

#1. Refined Sugar

The top food that causes anxiety is refined sugar, which includes white table sugar, brown sugar, corn syrup, sucrose, fructose, and high-fructose corn syrup. When you have low levels of serotonin in the brain, you crave sugar.[24] While you may feel good during your five-minute sugar high, you quickly experience a crash, which can be accompanied by anxiety.

There is an incredible amount of data showing how refined sugar deteriorates our health, including our mental health. One study found that consumption of added refined sugars, particularly high-fructose corn syrup and sucrose, negatively impacts your metabolism and the function of your hippocampus, and even causes neuroinflammation.[25]

In a study published in the journal *Diabetologia*, researchers reported that when blood glucose levels are elevated, levels of brain-derived neurotrophic factor (BDNF) decrease. BDNF is a protein that encourages the growth of neurons. Decreased BDNF is linked to dementia, depression, and even type 2 diabetes.[26]

Research has established a correlation between increased sugar intake and anxiety. A 2008 study showed that rodents that binged on sugar displayed instant anxiety, signs of dependence, and opiate-like withdrawal. The researchers suggested that sugar binges may "activate neural pathways in a manner similar to taking drugs of abuse."[27] One study called sugar "more rewarding and attractive" than cocaine![28]

Sugary beverages have been associated with higher risk of depression or depressive symptoms.[29] Yet in Britain, adults consume approximately double, and in the U.S., triple, the recommended level of added sugar, with sweet foods and drinks contributing to three-quarters of their intake. Meanwhile, major depression is predicted to become the leading cause of disability in high-income countries by 2030.[30]

Some people, even experts, have been known to say, "All sugar is sugar." I will wholeheartedly debate this; it's common sense that eating a tablespoon of white sugar and eating a tablespoon of apple result in quite different effects on the body. A 2009 study supports this, demonstrating that rodents fed sucrose were more likely to show symptoms of anxiety than others fed honey, which is high in antioxidants.[31]

Fructose has also been shown to compromise cognitive abilities like learning and memory. A study by researchers at the University of California, Los Angeles, revealed that six weeks of taking a fructose solution (similar to soda) caused rodents to forget their way out of a maze, whereas those that ate a nutritious diet or consumed a high-fructose diet that included omega-3 fatty acids found their way out faster. The high-sugar diet without omega-3 supplementation caused insulin resistance, which in turn damaged communications between the brain cells that fuel learning and memory formation![32]

High-fructose corn syrup is a low-cost sweetener you'll find in everything from ketchup to candy and crackers. Consuming high-fructose corn syrup is the fastest way to develop obesity, anxiety, depression, and other health issues. It is involved in a vicious cycle, too: It begins when a cause like chronic stress and anxiety depletes the brain's reserves of dopamine (not sleeping properly, eating a poor diet, or adrenal fatigue will do the same). This leads us to eat a quick sugary snack to boost our energy, making matters worse. We crash after eating the sugar, then crave more sugar. Reduced dopamine is associated with obesity because of how it contributes to compulsive eating. High-fructose corn syrup can impair dopamine function, and reduced dopamine function has been implicated in anxiety and compulsive behaviors.[33]

The saddest part is that foods with high-fructose corn syrup are being fed to children, impairing their brain's ability to learn and remember. Soda is often made with high-fructose corn syrup or white sugar. Do whatever you need to do to phase soda out of your life. Try drinking kombucha instead for a sweet fizzy drink that's also rich in probiotics.

This information about sugar may seem familiar, but I invite you to consider doing something radical: Never eat refined sugar again. A commitment would mean it's not part of the foundation of your diet. If you do end up eating it here and there, then so be it. (Make sure to boost your intake of omega-3s, as this may be protective against the effects of sugar.) But don't go out of your way to pursue white sugar. Do not keep it in your home. There is no need for it. Cut refined sugar from your diet, and I promise you will start to feel better immediately. There is no place for it anymore in our world—especially when we're feeling anxious.

Sneaky Sugar

It is important to check ingredient labels to see what type of sugar is in a food. (In fact, it's never wise to eat anything these days without checking its ingredient label first.) Watch out for the following names for "sneaky sugars" on the ingredient label:

- *Sugars:* brown sugar, beet sugar, raw sugar, white sugar, white granulated sugar, organic white sugar, evaporated cane juice, muscovado, turbinado sugar, panela, rapadura

- *Syrups:* corn syrup, high-fructose corn syrup, golden syrup, molasses, caramel, corn sweetener, treacle

- *Any ingredient ending in "-ose,"* including fructose, glucose, maltose, sucrose, dextrose, galactose, lactose, mannose, saccharose

Sucrose, fructose, and glucose are not "bad," per se. In fact, you'll find these compounds naturally occurring in many fruits and vegetables. However, if you see these names on a product list, that means that the ingredient has been extremely refined and extracted. The only time you want to consume sucrose, glucose, or fructose is in their natural state.

#2. Bad Fats

There are good fats and there are bad fats. It's easiest to remember that almost all the foods that come straight from nature contain the good fats we need, foods like avocado, walnuts, and chia seeds, among others. Bad fats are mostly human-made, including those you find in fried food, fast food, and hydrogenated oils (trans fats). Saturated fats are mixed when it comes to health effects—more on that later!

Don't be fooled by the seemingly low prices on fried food and fast food; the true price of that cheap fast food gets expensive real fast. According to many studies, people who eat fast foods like hamburgers, hot dogs, pizza, and baked goods are more likely to develop depression—in fact, they are more than 51 percent more likely to do so, according to a 2012 study in the journal *Public Health Nutrition.*[34] Yes, I still want to enjoy French fries for the rest of my life, but I try to avoid fast-food joints that cook them in low-quality, toxic oils. I seek out higher-quality foods or make them myself at home. When I fill myself up on good fats, I don't crave the bad fats.

Hydrogenated fats are liquid vegetable oils that are made creamy when manufacturers convert fats through hydrogenation, the process of adding hydrogen to a liquid fat to turn it into a solid. While full hydrogenation has risks you would wish to avoid, you should be most concerned about *partially* hydrogenated oils, which are known as trans fats. These should be cut from your diet without hesitation. Hydrogenated oils/trans fats have been causally linked to increased depression and anxiety.[35]

Trans fats became common in the 1950s and are found in margarine, snack foods, chips, packaged baked goods like muffins and crackers, and oils used to fry fast food. They are such a threat to public health that in May 2018 the World Health Organization released a six-point plan, known by the acronym REPLACE, to remove them from the global food supply.[36] Consuming trans fats can increase your risk of depression by as much as 48 percent, according to a study published in *PLoS One*.[37]

Trans fats have an adverse effect on the brain and nervous system. When we eat trans fat, it is incorporated into brain cell membranes and alters the ability of neurons to communicate. This can diminish mental performance and might create a feeling of brain fog. There is a direct relationship between eating trans fats and mental health issues.[38]

I saved the worst for last: Bad fats have also been linked to murder. Yes, that's right, trans fats lead to so much inflammation in the brain that it creates an agitated mood and aggressive behavior. Mark Hyman, M.D., shared some disturbing research on his blog showing how homicide in the United Kingdom increased dramatically with increased consumption of linoleic acid–rich soybean oil. The same thing happened in the United States, Australia, Canada, and Argentina.[39] Interestingly, apparently homicide rates are also inversely related to seafood consumption— meaning, societies in which more seafood is consumed have lower homicide rates.[40] Dr. Hyman makes a good point that the fats people are eating today aren't the ones our ancestors ate. Human evolution occurred in an environment where seafood and wild animal fat were the predominant sources of dietary fat, rather than trans fats and fried food.

Saturated fats, like the ones found in deli meats, high-fat dairy, and butter can clog arteries and prevent blood flow to the brain—inhibiting it from optimal function. What's worse is when these bad fats are mixed with sugar! Studies have shown that a dietary pattern characterized by saturated fats and added sugars is consistently associated with higher anxiety levels. This is because the consumption of saturated fats, processed foods, and added sugar causes alterations in glucose, protein, and energy homeostasis, and increases in inflammatory cytokines and corticosterone (an adrenal hormone).[41]

Not all saturated (and unsaturated) fats are created equal, however. Research has shown that medium-chain saturated fats (MCSFs) and monounsaturated fatty acids (MUFAs) have health benefits not found in long-chain saturated fatty acids (LCSFAs). LCSFAs promote insulin resistance, inflammation, and fat storage. MCSFs and MUFAs, on the other hand, are more likely to be burned for energy rather than stored as fat (adipose). Furthermore, omega-6 polyunsaturated fatty acids (PUFAs) may contribute to obesity, whereas omega-3 PUFAs may be protective.[42]

Most foods contain a combination of several types of fats, but the following foods are particularly rich in these fats:

- MCSFs: coconut oil

- MUFAs: olive oil, avocados, nuts, seeds

- LCSFAs: cream, butter, margarine, palm oil

- Omega-6 PUFAs: vegetable oils

- Omega-3 PUFAs: fish oils

Do not try to avoid fats altogether! Healthy fats have a purpose in our bodies: They metabolize fat-soluble nutrients so that our brains can function properly. When you avoid fats entirely, you ruin your health. You can experience burnout—complete exhaustion—and this leads to craving fast food and fried food. Stay nourished by healthy fats and the other stuff will be less appealing to you. Healthy fats also will reduce your inflammation. Replace bad fats with healthy fats like the following:

- Olives and olive oil
- Coconuts and coconut oil
- Raw nuts, such as macadamias and pecans
- Seeds, such as sesame, pumpkin, hemp, and chia
- Organic egg yolks from pastured poultry
- Meat from grass-fed, pasture-raised animals
- Butter or ghee made from raw, grass-fed, organic milk
- Animal-based omega-3 fat, such as krill oil
- Wild-caught salmon
- Cacao butter

Make sure to read all the ingredient labels for sneaky bad fats; you will be surprised where you find them. Even conventional nondairy creamers often use hydrogenated oils/trans fats.

#3. Toxic Chemicals Hidden as "Ingredients" in Food

Did you know that particular chemicals have been banned—for good reason—as food ingredients in many countries, yet the United States allows these same chemicals to be used in common foods we might eat every single day? They are banned in other countries because they are linked to countless health issues, including mental health issues and cancer. But in the U.S. they remain in foods because people continue to buy them and aren't speaking up about them. Nonetheless, the following should be avoided:

- Blue 1, Blue 2, Yellow 5, and Yellow 6: coloring agents found in anything fluorescent, like brightly colored candy, juices, cereal, and sauces
- Olestra (Olean): fat substitute found in some potato chips, French fries, corn chips, and other crunchy snack foods

- Potassium bromate (brominated flour): found in baked goods made with conventional white flour

- Azodicarbonamide (ADC): a bleaching agent found in baked goods made with conventional white flour

- Brominated vegetable oil (BVO): found in sodas and sports drinks

- Butylated hydroxyanisole (BHA) and butylated hydroxytoluene (BHT): found in packaged meat products, soup mixes, mayonnaise, and frozen meals

- Synthetic hormones (rBGH and rBST): found in dairy

- Diphenylamine (DPA): pesticide found on apples

We certainly do "vote" with our money. If we stop buying these foods, they will no longer be produced. I suggest that until the government sets higher standards for what foods are sold, we should all be mindful in who we support with our money and be wise in what we put in our mouths. It's going to require individual efforts on our own behalf to reduce our stress and anxiety, along with reducing it for people across the globe as a whole.

Many other toxic chemicals that are found in our foods can trigger immediate brain discord and anxiety:

- Pesticides and herbicides, including glyphosate: Pesticides contaminate most of our foods from any country using them, which definitely includes the United States, Australia, and the United Kingdom. Unfortunately, the United States is the top country in terms of heavy pesticide use.

- Polychlorinated biphenyls (PCBs) : found in pesticides used on crops

- Flame retardants: found in foods and also plastics, paint, furniture, and electronics

- Dioxins: found in meat and pesticides used on crops

- Phytoestrogens: found in soy and other foods

- Perfluorinated chemicals: they come from industrial processes and settle on crops

- Phthalates: found in food packaging and pharmaceuticals

- BPA (bisphenol A): found in canned foods and foods packaged in plastic. BPA has been exposed as neurotoxic in recent years, and that's why you will see so many canned foods and water bottles labeled "BPA free" now.

It's important to make sure that as many of your food sources as possible are organic and non-GMO. If the source is not organic, chances are that it is contaminated with pesticides, which can wreak havoc on the gut and brain. Most nonorganic wheat, for example, is treated with glyphosate, an herbicide shown to cause nutrient deficiencies—so much so that some scientists are "urging governments globally to reexamine the policy toward glyphosate and introduce new legislation that would restrict its usage."[43]

A Note about the Soil on Our Farms

We must be interested in where and how our food is being grown. We don't want to eat foods that are grown right next to big factories that are producing huge amounts of pollution, for this goes into the soil and depletes it of vital nutrients needed to grow nourishing foods. We also want the water supply that irrigates the crops to be clean and uncontaminated by chemicals from industrial runoff.

Our soils have become contaminated with pesticides and other toxic chemicals, making it even more important to buy organic fruits and vegetables. The soil on organic farms must meet certain requirements to keep it free from chemical alteration.

Polycyclic aromatic hydrocarbons (PAHs) have been found in soils that grow foods, and they accumulate in the soil. PAHs are naturally produced by forest fires and volcanoes. But most are emitted by coal gasification plants, smokehouses, motor vehicle exhaust, burning refuse and used tires, municipal incinerators, and some aluminum production facilities—as well as in facilities that are part of industries that produce or use coal tar, coke, or bitumen (asphalt). The food grown in these soils is extremely poor-quality, with contamination levels that can lead not only causes cancer but also mental health issues.

The constitution of the World Health Organization states, "Health is a state of complete physical, mental, and social well-being and not merely the absence of disease or infirmity."[44] This definition may sound exaggerated, but we must give up the foods mentioned in this chapter in order to gain real control over our brains, nervous systems, and guts. Eliminating them from our diets will lead to important health improvements and longevity.

#4. Artificial Ingredients: Sweeteners, Additives, Flavorings

Artificial sweeteners include aspartame (e.g., NutraSweet and Equal), saccharin (e.g., Sweet'N Low), and sucralose (e.g., Splenda). Aspartame, which is often found in diet soda and chewing gum, inhibits the synthesis and release of neurotransmitters, including dopamine, norepinephrine, and serotonin. It can also elevate plasma cortisol levels and cause the production of excess free radicals. This may lead to learning problems, headaches, seizures, migraines, irritable moods, anxiety, depression, and insomnia.[45] One study reported that a patient's movement consisted of rhythmic contractions of the arms and legs that were triggered by aspartame.[46]

Artificial flavoring and color seem to exacerbate behavioral issues, especially in children with ADHD, autism, and hyper-activity.[47] Yet artificial colors are found in unexpected places, including children's vitamins!

You will find toxic preservatives such as BHT and BHA, which are also found in dry cleaning solvent, in many processed foods in order to extend their shelf life.

MSG (monosodium glutamate) is a food additive used to enhance flavor. It is strongly associated in people's minds with

Asian take-out foods; however, its use is widespread. It's also found in canned soups and vegetables and processed meats.

You might also see MSG listed in an ingredient list as glutamate, glutamic acid, hydrolyzed protein or yeast extract, autolyzed yeast, or ingredient E621. Some companies even sneak it into the ingredient list under the term "natural flavors"!

MSG is classified as a food ingredient that's "generally recognized as safe" (GRAS), but it is incredibly controversial, and for a good reason. Although glutamate is a chemical that can naturally be found in some cheeses and vegetables, intake of MSG has been associated with psychological symptoms, including anxiety, but its effect can be much worse. At the extreme, it is linked to severe, chronic psychiatric disorders, including psychosis and depressive disorders.[48] In a study of healthy young adults, daily MSG intake over five days induced muscle pain and increased reports of headache.[49]

Artificial sweeteners, additives, and flavorings are neurotoxic, and yet they are found in both foods and food supplements. You will find artificial ingredients in many packaged foods and processed foods. Shockingly to me, even products that are meant to improve our health may contain them, including vitamins and supplements—even those meant for our children. How offensive!

#5. Refined Carbohydrates

Simple carbs, also known as simple sugar or refined carbs, are found in processed foods like cakes, cookies, breakfast cereal, pizza, and pastries. They should be avoided as much as possible, for the rest of your life. (Don't worry: I'll show you in the next chapter how you can still enjoy these things but in an "upgraded" way.)

Refined carbohydrates are made from wheat, which is fine in a balanced, healthy diet for some people; however, most processed carbs are made from low-quality wheat that has been genetically modified and grown in poor soil, saturated with pesticides, and then mixed with refined sugars to make a "food" like a cake or a bagel. The bottom line is that neurotoxic refined carbs include most sugars, trans fats, and processed grains.

Refined carbs may give you an initial surge of energy, but this can be followed by an insulin rush, which rapidly drops blood sugar levels, ultimately leaving you feeling lethargic. Substantial fluctuations in blood sugar can cause an immediate anxiety response in the body.

For example, a study was done with a 15-year-old female who presented concerns of generalized anxiety disorder and hypoglycemia symptoms. Her diet consisted primarily of refined carbohydrates. Protein, fat, and fiber were then added to her diet, a step that resulted in a substantial decrease in her symptoms of anxiety. A brief return to her previous diet caused a return of her anxiety, followed by another improvement when she restarted the prescribed diet.[50]

No need to be afraid of all carbohydrates, though; there are good and bad carbs. It's easiest to remember that good carbohydrates come from nature in whole foods like fruits, vegetables, and whole grains. Bad carbs come from human-made foods like bread, cakes, cookies, and muffins.

The good carbohydrates that you can eat as part of a balanced diet are oats, organic non-GMO wheat, and vegetables. If you want to eat things like muffins and cookies, check out my recipes in Part II of this book, which use alternative ingredients like almond flour, tigernut flour, and tapioca to make delicious, soft, and moist cakes.

Another helpful thing to remember is the principle of simple carbs versus complex carbs. Simple carbohydrates are found in foods such as milk, dairy products, pasta, sugar, white bread, and some fruits and vegetables. They are also found in processed and refined sugars like white sugar, syrups, and soft drinks.

Not all simple carbohydrates are bad, however. Fruits and vegetables may contain simple carbohydrates, but because they contain dietary fiber and are rich in micronutrients, such as vitamins and minerals, they may be considered healthful. If you need a quick sugar rush, it's better for you to get it from an apple than candy, which doesn't have those similar nutrients.

Complex carbs last longer in the body than simple carbs because they have more substantial molecules. They are called *complex* because they are made up of chains of three or more sugar molecules. Simple carbs, by contrast, contain only one or two sugar molecules. Beans, peas, whole grains (for instance, quinoa and rice), and vegetables are made up of complex carbohydrates.

Both simple and complex carbohydrates are turned to glucose (blood sugar) in the body and are used as energy. Complex carbs are high in fiber and take longer for your body to process, so they're more filling. Simple carbohydrates are broken down quickly to be used as energy. (This is why the body gets a quick sugar rush when you eat candy.) Eating simple carbs can cause major swings in blood sugar levels and contribute to impulse eating, binge eating, and overeating. They are also high on the glycemic index, providing short-term fullness. Complex carbs, in comparison, are a long-term fuel source.

Uma Naidoo, M.D., a nutritional psychiatrist and contributor to the *Harvard Health Blog*, explains how complex carbohydrates are metabolized more slowly and, therefore, help maintain a more even blood sugar level, which creates a calmer feeling. She says: "A diet rich in whole grains, vegetables, and fruits is a healthier option than eating a lot of simple carbohydrates found in processed foods. When you eat is also important. Don't skip meals. Doing so may result in drops in blood sugar that cause you to feel jittery, which may worsen underlying anxiety."[51]

#6. Processed Meat

Processed meat such as hot dogs, sausages, and meat pies can cause anxiety immediately after it's eaten! Researchers in London found that eating a diet of processed meats and fatty foods increased the risk of depression—in fact, the risk was 58 percent higher than for those who ate whole foods such as fish and vegetables.[52] We also need to be careful about nitrates, which are the chemicals used to cure processed meats. A study by Johns Hopkins Medicine found that rats fed a nitrate-rich diet showed mania-like hyperactivity after just a few weeks. The same researchers studied 1,000 people and found that those who had been hospitalized for mania had more than three times the odds of having eaten nitrate-cured meats than those without a history of a serious psychiatric disorder.[53]

If you want to eat sausages, try organic ones, made with healthy ingredients that won't destroy your brain.

#7. FARMED FISH

Farmed fish has become increasingly popular and doesn't sound nearly as harmful as it is. However, farm-raised salmon is nutritionally different from wild-caught salmon in a few ways. First, it has considerably more calories because of what it is fed. It is also much higher in fat, especially omega-6s, which can contribute to inflammation. Further, it is lower in minerals like potassium, zinc, and iron. Finally, and this is the main reason to avoid it, it is much higher in contaminants.[54]

Fish pick up chemicals such as dioxins and PCBs from the water they swim in. And they pick them up from the feed they are given, which in salmon farming often means grains grown with pesticides (hence the contamination). Fisheries also raise animals in crowded conditions, so they give the fish antibiotics to reduce the chance of infection. Everything they are exposed to is in their flesh.

* * *

There is a critical need to deliver better education to the public, physicians, and clinicians about the role of nutrients in sustaining mental health. More attention should be paid to diet therapy for the prevention and complementary treatment of anxiety and maintenance of mental wellness. The recipes in Part II were designed to have the therapeutic properties discussed in these chapters.

CHAPTER 5

The Food Upgrade Mindset for Living Anxiety-Free

Often when we feel anxious, we get the urge to eat something as a way of self-medicating. The trap we get into is eating the types of foods that make us feel worse, so we end up feeling even more anxiety! Many of us struggle today with *knowing* we shouldn't eat in a certain way because it does not help us heal and may even worsen our condition, but there is a part of us that still wants to eat that food, causing major internal conflict! This is one of those confusing human moments.

Fortunately, at the end of the day, we can laugh at it, although it may seem overwhelming while it's occurring. For me, the conflict ended with finding out I had a mass in my neck. This gave me the motivation to eat healthily. All I wanted to do to soothe my nerves was go out and eat some fried chicken and processed chocolate, but I saw that this would not make my situation any better. Assessing the seriousness of this conflict, I realized I had to figure out a way not to eat junk foods, or else I was probably going to make the cancer grow and spread.

Food upgrading or swapping is the concept that literally saved my life. I have lived it ever since; it stopped all of my cravings and impulses to eat unhealthy foods, and I am still indulging in the most delicious foods like fried chicken and fries, just in a completely brand-new way.

THE DEPRIVATION APPROACH VS. THE UPGRADE APPROACH

One approach some may try when a food craving hits is relying on willpower—just say no to every craving and impulse. In my experience working with clients and patients over the past decade, this deprivation approach isn't very realistic, especially for those who struggle with addiction and anxiety. They aren't able to say no all day—especially for the rest of their lives. I always ask my clients, "Do you think you will never eat a cookie again? Or some cake?" It's just not realistic!

People always fail at giving up bad foods with this approach. I did too. I would say to myself, "On Monday, I will start again, and I will never eat junk foods ever from then on." Then, Monday would come, and I would have a strong craving for gummy bears. I'd try to ignore it until the urge became so strong that I would give in and binge them. Deprivation backfires in a similar way for most people. God was leading me to something healthy and balanced that I could do for the rest of my life.

Food upgrading is it! After seeing thousands of people adopt this strategy over the past 10 years, I promise you that it can lead to the transformation of your body, mind, and spirit. Do not underestimate this approach because of its simplicity. It won't help you manage your anxiety if you eat foods that trigger chaos in your nervous system. Upgrading can bring you into a state of greater harmony and balance.

We can *strengthen* our bodies with nutrients while enjoying the flavors and textures we love from different foods. Because oftentimes, when we crave certain foods, like fried chicken, for example, it's a message that the brain is actually craving fat to support its functions. Or if you crave chocolate, it's a message that your body may be deficient in magnesium. So it's good to listen to your body and fulfill its needs with wholesome versions of its desires.

When I was working to restore my health and overcome the anxiety I felt, I got the idea to adopt this thought process: *Every time I am craving something to eat, I will find a way to eat it in the most natural way possible—in a way that nourishes my body and at the same time tastes really good.* I was immediately excited to try to find or invent new, healthier versions of the foods I loved. A huge burden was lifted from me. I felt lighter and more peaceful right away and thought, *Wow! Okay! I can eat chocolate for the rest of my life! But I have to find a way to do it with a chocolate that has cleaner ingredients.* It was a dream come true, because the item I craved most often was chocolate.

This was a decade ago, and there weren't as many organic choices available to us then. Although I did locate some organic chocolate in a health food store, which was an upgrade from conventional chocolate, it was sweetened with white sugar, an ingredient I wanted to avoid. So I started to make my own chocolate using cacao, almond flour, and honey. I would add peanut butter to make Chocolate Peanut Butter Balls! And I would eat up to 20 of them a day because, for me, this was a major improvement, an "upgrade" from the kind of chocolate I had formerly eaten in one day.

I was blown away by the flavor and texture! The result of making homemade chocolate was like a moist, buttery, delicious chocolate brownie—although it contained no gluten, no dairy, no soy, no preservatives, no GMO ingredients, and no refined sugar. It tasted absolutely delicious, all the while providing my body with protein, fiber, antioxidants, and other nutrients that were healthy and sustaining for my body. Discovering the food upgrade mindset was the best thing that ever happened to me!

When I am doing nutritional coaching, I always tell my clients: Start with your greatest obstacle food first. Replace that food, and the rest of the changes you want to make will be easier. It will also give you a lot of relief to move a huge rock from your path to wellness. For some people, the food blocking the path might be pizza, or pasta, or bread, or cheese, or candy. What is yours?

For years, chocolate was always my biggest weakness and the greatest obstacle to healthy eating.

Upgrading is how we can have our cake and eat it too! But— you get it—it has to be a *certain* type of cake for this to work.

I used the upgrade approach to replicate all my favorite foods. I made chicken nuggets with organic chicken and a coating of turmeric, almond flour, and sea salt. I made cheesecake with cashews. I made ice cream with almond milk. I used coconut oil instead of butter. I made cookie dough from almond flour and maple syrup. And I discovered that there is a healthier alternative for absolutely everything that we want to eat.

Upgrading means we can continue to eat the foods we love for the rest of our lives guilt-free! We can eat them and achieve optimal wellness.

Truly, it's worth repeating that it's not realistic for any of us to think, *I will start a new diet on Monday—after which I will never, ever eat cookies again.* We are not biologically programmed for deprivation. That's why millions of people are stuck in an "I'll start tomorrow" pattern. They are still eating junk food because that way will never work.

But when we adopt the approach of asking, *How can I eat cookies in a* healthy *way?* and then find a way to do so, we fulfill our cravings and have a pleasurable experience. Because this food tastes good and nourishes the body, it also leaves us with a sense of real satiety, and it calms our nervousness.

That's the key: Flood the body with nutrients at the same time that you are indulging in happiness-inducing, delicious flavors. It was mind-blowing for me to discover this. I wished I had learned it before I tried all those processed foods with refined sugars and become hooked on them.

If you get stuck and can't find an alternative to something you would like to eat, please let me know. So far, there hasn't been one food for which I haven't been able to find an upgrade that worked with someone's lifestyle and tastes. Tweet me @theearthdieter or send me a message via another social network, such as Facebook or Instagram (@TheEarthDiet). I would love to hear from you and help you upgrade your diet. I mean it! Nothing makes me happier than helping people find upgrades to foods that are damaging their bodies and causing anxiety.

THE UPGRADE THOUGHT PROCESS

When you have a craving, ask yourself: *How can I satisfy this in the best way possible?*

- *Worst-case scenario:* Low-quality, fast-food, and conventional options; GMO and nonorganic ingredients; high-sugar, high-fat foods; anything with artificial colors, flavors, and preservatives

- *Better upgrade:* The organic option with clean ingredients

- *Best upgrade:* Something you make yourself with the highest-quality ingredients you can buy

Let's say, for example, you want some French fries. The worst-case scenario is buying fries at a fast-food franchise made from GMO potatoes cooked in low-quality oil and seasoned with preservative-ridden salt. What is the upgrade in this situation?

The *better* version is to get them at an organic restaurant where the cook uses non-GMO potatoes and high-quality oil.

The *best* version is to cook them at home yourself. (In Part II, I have included a recipe for Cauliflower Cheese Fries, which are made with extra-virgin olive oil, baked in the oven rather than fried, and covered with a vegan "cheese" made of cauliflower.)

* * *

If you do opt for the worst-case scenario—perhaps because you're traveling and nowhere near an organic café or a kitchen— don't berate yourself for choosing that option. Guilt only increases stress. While eating, you can say to yourself, "I am choosing this food right now. I have control over it [say this even if you don't feel like you are in control], and I am in control of my next choice as well. I am committed to a healthy life. I am in the process of transforming my health and my food choices."

Furthermore, you can *upgrade the experience* by following the fries with Lemon Chlorophyll Water (see p. 168) or a freshly squeezed vegetable juice to assist with digestion and elimination of toxins. Your body will immediately feel less stress after consuming those foods.

Living the upgrade mindset reduces guilt. When you know you're moving toward health, even by a small, incremental step, you feel better and have more peace of mind. Plus, you feel way less deprived if you do the right thing. It's empowering!

Deprivation diets will only drive you crazy, leaving you feeling worse than when you started. It's important to be kind to yourself. Health is the goal—and feeling good and being at ease with yourself are indicators of good health. This is why upgrading is such a great tool.

When you want chocolate, eat chocolate. Just try to make sure it's organic. Organic cacao, which is an ingredient in chocolate, is featured in different recipes in this book. You can also have cheesecake, cupcakes, ice cream, mousse, burgers, burritos, fries— just upgrade them from the old familiar junk-food versions. There are recipes for all of these foods here as well.

When you upgrade, you're making a better choice. You're not sacrificing anything—except things that are harmful, like preservatives and additives that can trigger your feelings of anxiety. The result is that you're eating food that tastes amazing and provides your body with the nutrition it needs.

As I've said, I *love* eating dessert. Eating a lot of "upgraded" desserts contributed to my recovery from the tumor *and* makes me happy, which stops me from feeling anxious. If you have a sweet tooth like me, you'll be pleased to know that you can find almost anything to meet your sweet and creamy cravings in the dessert recipe section. Just follow the rule: Upgrade it. Make sure it is as natural as possible. The quickest upgrade decision is to choose organic ingredients.

EXAMPLES OF UPGRADES

The following upgrades will come up again and again. If you commit these to memory, you'll save yourself some time.

The Bread Upgrade: When you crave bread, get the highest-quality, freshly baked organic bread you can. If you're worried about the price difference, remind yourself that you are a high-quality person and you deserve high-quality foods that don't make you sick! Upgrade further by baking your own bread using organic, non-GMO ingredients.

The Salad Dressing Upgrade: When you're having salad, instead of using a premade, store-bought dressing filled with sugar and preservatives, choose an organic dressing. Upgrade further by making your own from simple ingredients like extra-virgin olive oil and lemon, or sesame oil and vinegar. (See "Make Your Own Homemade Salad Dressing . . . Forever!" on p. 208.)

The Burger Upgrade: When you crave a burger, get it from a restaurant that uses organic, free-range meat. Upgrade again by making your own burger at home. (Try the Grass-Fed Beef Burger on p. 231, the Chickpea Burger on p. 189, or its variation, the Bean Burger, with an organic ketchup.)

The Pizza Upgrade: When you're having a pizza, upgrade by buying it fresh from a pizza parlor that makes it with high-quality flour and cheese. There are also some great premade, organic pizzas available in health food stores these days, which makes our lives so much easier. You can get a pizza that's made with organic wheat and organic dairy, a gluten-free crust with organic dairy, or a gluten-free crust with vegan cheese. There are so many exciting options to try! Upgrade further by making it yourself with organic cheese and dough, topped with your favorite vegetables. (Try the Thai Chicken Pizza on p. 237.)

The Pasta Upgrade: You can upgrade pasta by eating varieties made from high-quality, organic, non-GMO flour. An even better upgrade is to make pasta dishes at home—try some of the new varieties made from chickpeas, lentils, black beans, mung beans, and edamame. Explore Cuisine is my favorite brand for this type of pasta—the different varieties taste amazing, and they are also great sources of protein and fiber. They're also gluten-free, meaning you can eat them without getting bloated. (See my recipes for Creamy, Delicious Vegan GF Mac 'n' Cheese on p. 191 and Walnut "Meatballs" with Zoodles on p. 187.)

The Salt Upgrade: Any salt that has fillers and anticaking preservatives is toxic for the body. Upgrade your salt by using pure sea salt. Salt is a beautiful, pure mineral and should have nothing else added to it.

The Oil Upgrade: Instead of using GMO vegetable oil (including plain "vegetable oil" and canola oil), use one of these non-GMO options: extra-virgin olive oil, extra-virgin coconut oil, avocado oil, hempseed oil, flaxseed oil, tigernut oil, sesame oil, almond oil, or chia seed oil. These are healthy oils for the body and brain.

The Dairy Upgrade: Make sure to upgrade your milk, yogurt, and cheese products to organic, non-GMO, hormone-free, antibiotic-free, and growth hormone–free (BGH-free) products from grass-fed, free-range cows—and sourced as locally as possible.

The Cheese Upgrade: If you are eating dairy cheese, make sure that it is organic and high-quality. For a vegan upgrade, make your own recipes with nutritional yeast. Nutritional yeast is a vegan's best friend!

The Flour Upgrade: If you want to make a recipe that calls for flour, you must absolutely go for organic flour; often flour is genetically modified and sprayed with a lot of pesticides and herbicides. For sure, you don't want those chemicals going into your body and messing up your nervous system and brain. For a gluten-free flour mix, these work really well: arrowroot, tapioca, brown rice flour, potato starch, and buckwheat.

The Egg Upgrade: Upgrade your eggs to organic, non-GMO, hormone-free, antibiotic-free, growth hormone–free eggs from pasture-raised, free-range chickens. Buy local, if possible.

The Fries Upgrade: When you crave French fries, get a batch from a café that uses high-quality oil. Upgrade further by making them at home using organic potatoes and extra-virgin coconut oil. (See Cauliflower Cheese Fries on p. 199.)

Chocolate Upgrade: When you crave chocolate, buy organic chocolate made from pure ingredients: no dairy, soy, preservatives, or refined sugar. Upgrade further by making your own raw chocolate at home. (See Chocolate SunButter Cups on p. 252, Chocolate Avocado Mousse on p. 249, and Genius Chocolate Balls on p. 246.)

The Potato Chip Upgrade: When you feel like eating chips or crisps, go for non-GMO, organic potato products. There are some excellent brands out there. Upgrade further with baked kale chips.

The Candy Upgrade: When you crave candy, get organic candy that is also free of corn syrup, gluten, gelatin, and preservatives. Upgrade further by dehydrating a fruit puree at home, which is squished into different shapes. (Try Fruit Leather on p. 258).

The Cookie Upgrade: Buy organic, non-GMO cookies with few, simple ingredients. Upgrade further by making your own. Even more of an upgrade is eating the nutrient-dense Smart Cookies (see p. 247), which is eggless and therefore safe to eat raw as well as in its baked variation. You can actually get vitamins and minerals from this! Yes, cookie dough *can* be brain food and help reduce anxiety.

The Soda Upgrade: Conventional soda is dangerous because it contains ridiculous amounts of GMO sugar, caffeine, preservatives, colorings, flavorings, additives, and aspartame. Upgrade with organic sodas made from honey and fruit, or try kombucha, which is a probiotic and aids digestion.

The Energy Shot Upgrade: Excessive reliance on caffeine can increase anxiety and cause adrenal burnout. Furthermore, many of the most popular brands of energy shots contain damaging chemicals. Upgrade with the Hotshot Citrus (see p. 160). Also seek out one of the new, more enlightened fruit-based energy shots made with yerba maté, stevia, and high levels of B vitamins (often these do also contain caffeine, so read the labels).

The Alcohol Upgrade: Avoid alcohol when you feel anxious. However, if you decide to drink, organic wines without sulfites, organic tequila, and organic vodka (especially potato vodka, as it is gluten-free) are your best, cleanest upgrades for alcoholic beverages. Use mixes that do not contain refined sugar or corn syrup.

* * *

It's time to release any guilt you feel about your past food choices. Now that you know there are healthier alternatives, you can choose those instead! Remember what Maya Angelou says: "Do the best you can until you know better. Then when you know better, do better." Now you know.

When a craving hits, take a moment to remember the upgrade mindset. There is a healthy upgrade for every imaginable kind of craving—crunchy, sweet, creamy, savory, and salty. You will feel so nourished and be anxiety-free.

Also remember, organic vegetables and fruits don't need upgrades. Eat plenty every day! You really cannot go wrong by eating more and more vegetables.

ANXIETY-FREE WITH FOOD RECIPES

Welcome to the recipe section! Here you will find comfort food, which is what we need for the rest of our lives. But this isn't your typical comfort food. This comfort food is nourishing—meaning, it provides our brains with healthy fats, antioxidants, and energy!

Comfort foods provide a sense of consolation and a feeling of well-being—and even boost your serotonin levels.[1] Typically, they are high in sugar, but these particular recipes are sweetened naturally with fruits, honey, maple syrup, or coconut sugar. These are the healthy sugars your body can keep up with and that won't freak out your brain.

Comfort foods also are usually carbohydrates. There are plenty of healthy carbohydrates here that won't trigger a stress response in your body; they are vegetables and whole grains that your body will use as fuel.

Some of these recipes will remind you of cooking you ate in childhood, but with a healthy twist. So many great, whole-food ingredients can provide us with tastes, textures, and smells that are reminiscent of our favorite comfort foods from long ago. What is a life without comfort foods? Well it isn't really *living*, is it?

Here are the comfort foods you will find in Part II:

- Burgers: both plant-based (vegan) and beef

- Walnut-crusted chicken for your "fried chicken" cravings

- Potato lovers get cheese fries, mashed potatoes, French fries, and hash browns

- Pasta dishes

- Mac 'n' cheese

- Grilled cheese

- Chili

- Tomato soup

I am convinced everyone needs to be living a natural lifestyle like the Earth Diet, which means eating only foods made from ingredients that nature provides for us. If only we always fulfilled our cravings in this way, we would maintain healthy bodies for the rest of our lives! It's processed foods that cause all our health problems. I hope you will enjoy these recipes as much as I do, and that you will be able to enjoy them for many years to come.

The recipes are made of ingredients that are proven to boost the body's production of neurotransmitters, including plenty of fatty acids that play a critical role in brain health—both in the overall prevention of cognitive diseases and in reducing anxiety.

In conclusion, I believe that to reduce anxiety and help the body feel its best, aim for a diet rich in plants: vegetables, fruits, nuts, and seeds. To boost your protein, you can add small portions of carefully chosen fish, meat, poultry, and eggs. Think of the foods eaten in the Mediterranean, and then:

- Fill up on plenty of vegetables, nuts, seeds and fruits.

- Get your starch fix from whole grains and legumes.

- Focus on eating fatty fish like wild-caught salmon.

- Eat plenty of salads with homemade salad dressings made with extra-virgin olive oil, coconut oil, and nuts.

But what to do about sweets? We all know that eating sweets releases all these feel-good chemicals in our bodies momentarily. People of the Mediterranean enjoy sweets in moderation; however, this is where my approach differs from theirs. I don't believe in moderation for white table sugar. I believe in eating none! Why have any when we could have coconut sugar or honey instead? Especially when things taste just as good, if not better, made with unprocessed sweeteners. I can't stand the taste of white sugar now; it tastes so artificial and leaves a hollow, unfulfilled sensation in my mouth, body, brain, and gut.

I've experimented with eating a few things with white sugar over the years, and it's always an interesting experiment. It's amazing how much our taste buds change when we're consistent; we can create a new body based on these whole foods. White table sugar, even just a teaspoonful, will cause a crash in energy after making us feel temporarily high. The body experiences symptoms as a result of its attempts to digest the refined sugar, usually things like bloating, headaches, anxiety, and irritability.

The key is that we want to enjoy sweets that nourish the body and don't lead to a negative backlash. Refined sugar will only trigger anxiety, which means there is no place for white table sugar or corn syrup in our desserts. I say this strongly, because unfortunately refined sugar is destroying people's health.

Most of the dessert recipes are no-bake. They are raw and made just by adding some ingredients in a bowl or blender and mixing.

All of the recipes in this book are gluten-free. There are options to use a vegan cheese or dairy, if you do choose to have dairy because it works well for your body; just make sure it is the best quality you can get, organic, and non-GMO. Remember that you are a high-quality person and you want only the best going into your body and feeding your brain. These recipes use ingredients that the earth naturally provides and incorporate the least amount of processed ingredients possible.

Are you ready to eat your way to calm while gaining cognitive power? Let's do it!

CHAPTER 6

Kitchen Supplies and Conversion Charts

Many of the recipes in this book are so simple to make and eat that you'll often need just a bowl and a spoon. This is how food should be; the last thing we need to do right now is complicate things! Being anxiety-free is about getting back to basics and simplicity. The less time we spend confused about our food choices and making complex recipes, the more space we create in our minds.

In this recipe section of the book, I've got your back. You'll be able to make many of these recipes (and eat them) with your hands, like the Genius Chocolate Balls. You can also have peace of mind that this type of eating is quite like an ancestral diet. It's going back to nature . . . back to peace.

Some recipes will require you to use a juice machine and some a blender. Some are made on the stovetop and a few are baked. But many of these recipes are for raw dishes. By nature, just mixing raw ingredients like we do for the Genius Chocolate Balls is quick and produces food that is ridiculously high in nutrients.

Other special kitchen supplies for some of these recipes include:

- *Gummy bear molds:* To make Elderberry Gummy Bears, you will need gummy molds, which are likely easier to find online than in stores. Get some that are BPA-free.

- *Paper baking cups:* You will need these if you are going to make the Blueberry Muffins, Mini Cashew Cheesecakes, or Chocolate SunButter Cups. Look for FSC-certified compostable, unbleached, chlorine-free baking cups; they are better for the environment and your health than the standard type.

Kitchen Supplies

Here are the supplies you'll need to set up your anxiety-free kitchen! These would be the top three most important pieces of equipment to have if you must prioritize:

- Juice machine
- High-speed blender/food processor
- Teflon-free cookware

If you asked me, "What is the number one thing I need in my kitchen to live an anxiety-free life?" I would say:

"A JUICE MACHINE to make juices!" If this is the only appliance you have, well, at the very least you are getting a huge daily dose of vitamins and live enzymes by making your own homemade juices. Having one juice a day is everything, as I talked about in more detail in the previous chapters.

There are two types of juicers you'll generally encounter:

- *Regular juice machines:* Standard juicers have blades to chop up the produce inside, then use centrifugal force to separate the juice from the pulp. The process heats up the juice, which may affect nutrients and enzymes. Prices of models start from around $40, and you can get a good one for $100 to $200. This is all you may need for five years or so. This juice should be drunk the day it is made.

- *Masticating juicers:* Usually referred to as "slow" or cold-press juicers, these machines exert a pressing force on the produce you put into them instead of just giving you a lot of speed like a regular juicer, in order to limit the amount of heat created and thus preserve the nutritional value of the juice. These machines are generally pricier than centrifugal ones. Juice made from a centrifugal machine should be drunk the day it is made. By contrast, the nutrients in a juice made with a high-quality cold-press machine can stay intact for up to five days.

Here are a couple things that you should look for in a juicer:

- Stainless-steel construction: These machines have proven to be the best quality.

- Wide chute, capable of juicing whole apples: This will save you time by not having to cut up fruits and vegetables.

I used to recommend everyone get a juice machine and then also a separate blender to make smoothies, but then I discovered the Nama juicer. This is a blender and juice machine in one! You can use it to make juices, smoothies, nut milks, and even sorbet. The juices and nut milks that come out taste absolutely divine. Because the Nama is a cold-pressing "slow" juice machine, your ingredients aren't zapped with a lot of electricity (as happens with many other juicers) and the nutrients are left intact. You can definitely taste the difference.

It's worth investing in your juice machine and blender (or an appliance that combines both!) because this will be your daily dose of food-medicine. This is an investment in your health. They can run on the expensive side, but please don't let the price stop you. Payment plans are often an option. Some people say to me, "But it's so much cheaper for me to eat fast food." Well, it's really not! You pay for it in another way, as it affects your brain and every cell in your body.

A HIGH-SPEED BLENDER like the Vitamix is essential to make raw desserts, sauces, and more. A powerful blender with a reliable motor and sharp stainless-steel blades will work. If you have a strong enough blender, you won't need a food processor for these recipes. In general, blenders are better for wet mixtures, while a food processor is better for dry ingredients like making an almond meal.

I use a Vitamix blender because this is how I achieve creamy and ridiculously delicious smooth desserts like Cashew Ice Cream Bites, Mini Cashew Cheesecake, Chocolate Avocado Mousse, and Chocolate Sauce. Cheaper blenders with flimsy blades won't make a nut meal, so it's best to invest in a high-quality machine and have that for years and years. I know some people who have had their Vitamix for 20 years! No other machine in the world really compares for whipping up things to be so decadent and creamy. If you want to make homemade ice cream, this is the appliance to get.

QUALITY COOKWARE is so important to have—make sure the material is lead-free and nonreactive to the foods you cook in it, like stainless-steel, ceramic, and glass. My personal preference is stainless steel. The pots for cooking have thick bottoms. Ultimately, slow heating, as you would use when cooking on a fire or over coals, is the most natural form of cooking. Stay away from flimsy pots or nonstick pots and pans coated with Teflon and other synthetic materials. According to experts I trust, once heated these can spoil the food and become toxic. Of particular concern is the damage they may do to the immune and nervous systems.

Teflon nonstick coating may sound appealing and convenient, but it's really dangerous in the long run. Teflon is made from perfluorooctanoic acid (PFOA), which was shown to cause oxidative stress and inflammation, two causative factors in anxiety, in a rodent study.[1] PFOA is also found in microwave popcorn bags and carpet. There have been so many studies on the adverse effects of this substance, and PFOA was found in the blood of an estimated 98 percent of Americans![2] Can you believe it? This is crazy!

Removing all the things in your entire home that cause oxidative stress can be helpful in preventing and healing anxiety, which is why it's important to switch your foods and kitchen utensils to be as safe as possible. Throw out your Teflon-coated pots and pans if you can; they are not safe! But don't stress. Everything is a process. Just make sure you are in action and moving forward the best you can.

A few more kitchen essentials can make your cooking life much easier:

- A 12-inch-diameter stainless-steel skillet
- A large stainless-steel baking sheet
- A stainless-steel pot (six to eight cups)
- A stainless-steel or glass mixing bowl (six to eight cups)

UTENSILS will also be helpful (make sure they're BPA-free and nontoxic):

- A large spoon
- A sharp all-purpose knife for cutting and chopping
- A bamboo or wood cutting board
- A set of measuring cups
- A set of measuring spoons

A FOOD DEHYDRATOR is helpful if you want to make dried fruit and fruit leathers for roll-ups and candy. You can even dry your own herbs! If you don't have a dehydrator, you can use your oven; however, this isn't ideal as your oven would be on for several hours. This a bonus kitchen item—it's not a must-have like the juice machine. It is really fun and rewarding to make your own dried fruit and crackers!

A Few Special Ingredients in the Recipes Worth Mentioning

In case you are wondering about the ingredients in the recipes to come, you should stock your pantry with:

- *Avocado oil.* This is an oil option that is healthy to cook with, including for frying and baking. Some avocado oils have high heat points, up to 500°F, which makes them excellent for frying.

  It's particularly important to stick with a trusted brand of avocado oil. A study in 2020 by researchers from the University of California, Davis, discovered that 82 percent of the brands they tested were rancid or adulterated with other oil. Three avocado oils labeled "pure" or "extra virgin" were found to be nearly 100 percent soybean oil![3] That's why I recommend Nutiva brand oil, which is one of the few organic avocado oils available.

- *Coconut oil, butter flavored.* Nutiva butter-flavored coconut oil is a staple in my kitchen, so you'll see that a lot of my recipes are made with it. It is my go-to alternative to butter, as it has a buttery flavor and smell. Personally, I don't do well with intake of any dairy, so this is an excellent alternative for me. If you enjoy butter, you may use it in recipes that call for this ingredient; however, please just make sure your butter is grass-fed organic butter. Nutiva's buttery coconut oil is made from coconut oil, annatto (a seed), and fermented mint.

- *Liquid amino acids.* Amino acids are organic compounds from protein. With respect to these recipes, I am referring to either a salty-tasting organic soy sauce that contains amino acids or non-salty coconut amino acids (soy-free). So you can use either; it's up to you if you want to be soy-free. Personally,

I will eat some soy every now and then, but it must be non-GMO. I customarily use Bragg Liquid Aminos because this brand offers both types of amino acids.

- *MCT oil.* MCT oil is coconut oil that has gone through a refinement process that involves extracting and isolating the medium-chain triglycerides. The reason people are manufacturing this product now is because it contains more caprylic acid—a compound that energizes the brain—than regular coconut oil. MCT is also said to be more easily absorbed into the digestive system. MCT oil is a liquid, not a hard-set coconut oil. I use it as a booster in recipes for smoothies, soups, and desserts. It also makes a great base for salad dressing. If you don't have MCT oil on hand, you can use coconut oil instead; it just won't provide the same benefits and the result will be thicker in consistency.

- *Organic plant protein.* Look for a high-quality brand that's organic, non-GMO, low sugar, and low carb. I use Nutiva brand organic plant protein powder in smoothies and when baking items like muffins. I favor this product for many reasons. It's vegan, loaded with superfood ingredients, and absolutely delicious. I also trust the quality of it.

  A note on rice: Have a look at the ingredient list of many protein powders, and you'll find that they are generally rather high in carbs. This is often because the manufacturers add sugars or rice to them. Rice is a common, unnecessary, cheap filler. If we want rice, we should eat it whole, not in a protein powder.

- *Sea salt.* Table salt is toxic for us; real salt is an essential mineral that is vital for the human body. Too much salt mineral, or too little, is not healthy, so we need to find a healthy balance. Table salt usually contains anticaking agents, which we want to avoid.

I use Redmond Real Salt, which is ideal if you live in the United States, as it's local to us because it comes from Redmond, Utah. I've been to the salt mine where this is sourced, and it was amazing to see firsthand where it comes from. The land the mine is on was covered by the same ocean that covered the Himalayan mountains 2 million years ago. Real Salt is a light-pink color, courtesy of its unique mineral content. Redmond is a big family-run business, and there are good people behind it. They also make the bentonite clay that I speak of often, as there are natural clay deposits right next to the salt mine.

An alternative for Real Salt is Celtic Sea Salt, which comes from France. Celtic Sea Salt is a coarser salt that's good for cooking meat.

You can also use Himalayan salt. This pink salt technically is "sea salt" too.

Whatever you choose, keep in mind that it may have to be shipped to you, which can be quite taxing on the environment. It is best to use the salt that is sourced closest to you.

- *Sunflower seed butter.* My favorite brand, SunButter, makes several sunflower seed butters. I recommend it for many of my recipes, but please make sure you're using a non-GMO, organic sunflower butter, not a butter that contains sugar or is not labeled "organic." The SunButter organic sunflower butter is made from just one ingredient: roasted sunflower seeds. Not all the company's sunflower farms are certified organic. (I went and visited their farm to see for myself, and it's amazing!)

  SunButter has a texture similar to peanut butter and tastes like a cross between tahini and peanut butter. It's free of the top allergens, so it's great for anyone who has a nut allergy. I also love

SunButter because when I was eating so many nuts, I needed something to balance that out. I wanted to incorporate more seeds in my diet, especially sunflower seeds, as they provide vitamin E that is good for the skin and they are incredibly high in antioxidants.

This butter makes a great snack. If you ever feel anxious, just have a spoonful of SunButter or put some on an apple or carrot. It's also a great nutrient booster in smoothies and in savory recipes, especially Asian-style dishes like pad thai or satay noodles. You can use this as a substitute in any recipe that calls for peanut butter, since sunflower seed butter ticks more of the antianxiety boxes when compared to peanut butter.

- *CBD oil.* If CBD is part of your anxiety-free plan, you can add it to most of these recipes, especially the desserts. Just add it to the blender or bowl when mixing. For example, you might swirl a serving (see product label and packaging materials for appropriate dosage) into the Cashew Ice Cream Bites with Chocolate Sauce or the Genius Chocolate Balls. It's also great to add to smoothies. And if you want to cook with CBD, combine it with the oils so that it binds well and will distribute into the food.

- *Gluten-free flours.* I often use potato starch and tapioca flour (also known as tapioca starch) as a thickening agent in my recipes instead of cornstarch, which may be made from GMO corn. Tapioca flour, which is extracted from cassava (yucca) root, also makes an epic gluten-free flour for baking. I also like baking with almond flour and tigernut flour.

METRIC CONVERSION TABLE
(MEASUREMENTS AND TEMPERATURES)

If you adhere to the metric system, the chart at the end of the book can help you convert the quantities of ingredients in the Anxiety-Free with Food recipes from ounces and pounds to grams and kilos. Find it on p. 275.

> Go to **LianaWernerGray.com** for recommendations and coupon codes on equipment and kitchen supplies I believe are the healthiest and most effective. Come back and visit regularly—the list of products and discounts is always evolving as I continue to search for new ways to make our lives easier, more time efficient, and healthier.

CHAPTER 7

Brain-Boosting Drinks

Liquids are a great way to put nutrition straight into your system. Think of drinking a juice or smoothie as being like an IV, where you can get a cocktail of vitamins pumped directly into your system through a needle. Liquids are an easily absorbed, natural way to get a vitamin boost.

Starting every day with a glass of lemon water and a few drops of chlorophyll is powerful. Any leafy green ingredient you put into a juice will give you a dose of chlorophyll without the need for supplementation. (Remember that chlorophyll is what gives those plants a vibrant green color.)

Here you will discover undiluted juices made from fresh fruits and vegetables of all different colors. These are considered raw meals or drinks. The key nutrients that give raw juices tremendous brain-boosting power are flavonoids and antioxidants. Colorful produce is loaded with both.[1]

Smoothies are a great way to pack a meal into a cup. They can be high in protein—I often get mine up to 30 grams of protein with the inclusion of a plant-based protein powder, SunButter, kale, and spinach. This is very satiating, and you can make your smoothie in the range of 200 to 500 calories for a meal if you want.

The difference between a shake and a smoothie is that a smoothie is thick, with an ice cream–like consistency, whereas a shake is light, like a milk. If you are feeling hungrier, go for a smoothie and pack it with a protein powder and boosters to feed your brain. Shakes are lighter and usually fewer calories, so make one of those if you aren't as hungry and yet want a nutrient hit.

Smoothies are thicker than juices, while offering the same range of antioxidants and phytonutrients from fresh produce with more fiber remaining. They can be sweet or savory.

Teas can be a great way to start and end the day. They are soothing during the middle of the day, as well, if you need a tea break. The teas here are high in antioxidants, providing you with some energy, switching on your brain, and at the same time relaxing your nervous system.

Cleansing waters are simply a water with an infusion of lemon or other fruit to provide additional health benefits.

Elixirs are a particular type of medicinal solution. The ones you see here are specifically designed for reducing anxiety, as they use particular herbs and flowers.

Smoothie Tips

- To make it sweeter, add seeded dates or honey.

- Use frozen cauliflower rather than fresh—raw cauliflower adds too much flavor. Frozen cauliflower helps make a thick, creamy smoothie.

- For a low- to no-sugar smoothie, substitute frozen cauliflower for any fruits.

- If you don't want to use frozen cauliflower, substitute banana or other fruits.

- Add a serving of reishi mushrooms for more neuroprotective benefits. (Dose depends on whether it's in capsule, liquid, or powder form—see label for instructions.)[2]

- For additional health benefits, add a serving of bee pollen.[3]

SUPER GREENS JUICE

As I previously mentioned, I have committed to one green drink every single day for the rest of my life, whether it is a green juice, green smoothie, or chlorophyll water. I believe it is important to maintain optimal health. It is my mission to help others commit to this also. If this were the only healthy thing you ever did, you would be much better off. And when people ask me what I recommend they do if they can change only one thing—this is it.

You can get all your essential greens from one drink with this recipe, which combines several of the top anxiety-reducing foods, like the dark leafy greens, ginger, and lemon!

Total time: 10 minutes • Makes 1 serving

Ingredients:

1 cucumber

1 green apple or ¾ cup pineapple

3 celery stalks

½ cup kale

½ cup spinach

1 cup broccoli sprouts

1 handful of fresh parsley

½ lemon, peeled

1 thumb-size piece of ginger

Actions:

Juice all the ingredients in your juicer and drink.

If you want a sugar-free juice, make this recipe without the apple (or pineapple). This is something I do often.

BEET JUICE

Beets are great digestive cleansers. This juice not only detoxifies the blood and liver, it also helps lift compacted waste from the bowel wall, which will enable your bowels to absorb brain-healthy nutrients more effectively.

Beets help soothe anxiety in another way, too. They are a source of nitrate, and thus increase the level of nitric oxide in our blood. This means beets relax the inner muscles of the blood vessels, which increases our blood flow while lowering our blood pressure. Beets also help reduce inflammation and oxidative stress.[4]

Total time: 10 minutes • Makes 1 serving

Ingredients:

1 small beet

1 red apple

3 carrots

2 celery stalks

½ small lemon, peeled

1 thumb-size piece of ginger

Actions:

Juice all the ingredients in your juicer and drink.

Tip:

Replace the apple with carrots for less sweetness.

VITAMIN C BLAST

The delicious blend of vibrant citruses in this beverage will uplift your mood. Studies have shown that eating orange, lemon, and grapefruit can help relieve anxiety, and so can just the scent of them![5] So make sure to inhale the aroma of the ingredients when you make this juice.

One of the best things about this recipe is that you can squeeze the juice by hand, either with a hand juicer or your own bare hands, which is a way to relieve some stress and practice calming mindfulness. Bonus: This combination is a sweet way to blast away excess fat cells.

Total time: 10 minutes • Makes 1 serving

Ingredients:

2 oranges, peeled

1 grapefruit, peeled

½ lemon, peeled

Dash of turmeric powder

Actions:

1. Juice all the ingredients in your juicer or squeeze them by hand.
2. Add a small sprinkle of turmeric powder, stir, and drink.

ORANGE CARROT GINGER JUICE

Carrots are an important root vegetable that is rich in carotenoids, anthocyanins, dietary fiber, vitamins, and other nutrients. Carrots serve as sources of antioxidants and have important functions in preventing many diseases.[6] They also help make our skin glow from the inside out, a great way to keep a "tan" even during the winter months. (But don't worry—it would take consuming six carrots a day for six months for your skin to start turning orange.)

Total time: 10 minutes • Makes 1 serving

Ingredients:

1 orange, peeled

4 carrots

1 thumb-size piece of ginger

Actions:

Juice all the ingredients in your juicer and drink.

MASTER SMOOTHIE

This is the smoothie I drink the most! It's called the master because it contains multiple brain-boosting superfoods and also takes the prize for being a nutritional powerhouse with its combination of greens, omega-3 fatty acids, and plant-based protein. Out of all the smoothies I recommend, this one has the highest amount of protein: 29 grams per serving. I really hope you try this masterpiece—a divinely creamy, icy, and refreshing smoothie that will keep your brain satiated for hours. This makes a great meal replacement.

Total time: 10 minutes • Makes 1 serving

Ingredients:

1 cup hemp milk or coconut milk
¾ frozen banana
½ cup ice
2 tablespoons organic SunButter or almond butter
½ teaspoon spirulina
1 handful of spinach or kale

1 scoop Nutiva vanilla-flavored plant protein (or any protein powder made from anything but rice)
½ teaspoon flax meal or seeds
1 teaspoon MCT oil

Actions:

Blend all the ingredients in a blender until the mixture reaches a smooth consistency. Pour into a glass, drink, and enjoy!

GREEN GODDESS SMOOTHIE

Feel like a goddess instantly while drinking this vibrant and refreshing green smoothie.

Total time: 10 minutes • Makes 1 serving

Ingredients:

1 cup coconut milk or macadamia nut milk

1 scoop Nutiva vanilla-flavored plant protein, or another plant-based protein powder

¼ cup frozen mango

¼ cup frozen pineapple

¼ cup spinach

¼ cup kale

1 tablespoon tigernuts or almonds

1 tablespoon almond butter

½ teaspoon chlorella or spirulina

½ teaspoon flax meal or seeds

½ teaspoon chia seeds

Actions:

Blend all the ingredients in a blender until the mixture reaches a smooth consistency. Pour into a glass, drink, and enjoy!

Tip:

For extra creaminess and healthy fats, add ½ avocado.

GENIUS SMOOTHIE

You'll see why it's called the Genius Smoothie after you have the experience of feeling focused, sharp, and energized for hours after drinking it! Packed with all the brain's favorite superfoods, this smoothie has so many immune-boosting elements to it.

Total time: 10 minutes • Makes 1 serving

Ingredients:

½ frozen banana

⅓ cup frozen blueberries

1 cup hemp milk

½ cup ice

1 scoop Nutiva chocolate-flavored MCT powder

1 tablespoon almond butter

1 teaspoon maca

¼ cup spinach

1 tablespoon walnuts

½ teaspoon spirulina powder

1 teaspoon flax meal or flax oil

1 teaspoon hempseeds

½ teaspoon chia seeds

Actions:

Blend all the ingredients in a blender until the mixture reaches a smooth consistency. Pour into a glass, drink, and enjoy!

Tip:

Add 1 serving size of powdered reishi mushrooms for more neuro-protective benefits.

CHOCOLATE SUPREME

By now, you know how powerful cacao is and that it is a functional food that promotes optimum brain and gut health. Bonus: It tastes like dessert. Wow, life is good!

Total time 10 minutes • Makes 1 serving

Ingredients:

1 cup almond milk

½ cup ice

½ frozen banana

½ cup frozen cauliflower

2 tablespoons frozen blueberries

2 tablespoons almond butter, peanut butter, or organic SunButter

1 teaspoon cacao nibs

1 teaspoon maca powder

½ teaspoon flax oil

Actions:

Blend all the ingredients in a blender until the mixture reaches a smooth consistency. Pour into a glass, drink, and enjoy!

Tip:

For a caramelly, nutty flavor, add a serving of mesquite powder.

CHOCOLATE TIGERNUT BERRY SMOOTHIE

I drank this smoothie every day for a solid year! It helped restore my brain so much, while at the same time tasting absolutely delicious.

Total time: 10 minutes • Makes 1 serving

Ingredients:

2 cups frozen berries of your choice (strawberries, raspberries, and/or blueberries)

2 tablespoons almond butter

1 cup Nut-Free Tigernut Milk (see p. 163)

1 tablespoon (or more) cacao powder

1 tablespoon raw honey

Actions:

Blend all the ingredients in a blender until the mixture reaches a smooth consistency. Pour into a glass, drink, and enjoy.

HOTSHOT CITRUS

Total time: 10 minutes • Makes 1 serving

Ingredients:

2 oranges, peeled

1 grapefruit, peeled

½ lemon, peeled

1 thumb-size piece of ginger

Dash of turmeric powder

Actions:

Add all the ingredients to a blender and mix until well combined. Pour into a glass, drink, and enjoy!

BASIC NUT MILK AND SEED MILK FORMULA

With this basic formula, you can make your own plant-based milk for the rest of your life. To make a gallon of milk, you'll need to quadruple the recipe. This milk (as well as the coconut, oat, and tigernut milk recipes on the next pages) can be kept in the refrigerator for up to a week, or frozen in airtight containers for a month or more.

Total time: 5 minutes • Makes 4 servings

Ingredients:

1 cup raw nuts or seeds of your choice (see options below)

4 cups filtered water

⅛ teaspoon vanilla extract

3 seedless dates (or 1 to 2 tablespoons raw honey or maple syrup)

Dash of sea salt

Nut Options:

Almonds

Brazil nuts

Cashews

Hazelnuts

Macadamia nuts

Seed Options:

Hempseeds

Flaxseeds

Sunflower seeds

Actions:

Put all the ingredients in a high-speed blender, and mix until a smooth consistency is achieved. Pour into a glass to drink immediately, or place in a covered container for storage in the refrigerator or freezer.

Tips:

- If your blender is not very powerful, you can soften your nuts by soaking them in water for 4 hours or overnight. Drain and discard the soaking water before adding the nuts to your blender.

- You can strain the milk through cheesecloth or another fine cloth, if necessary, to achieve a smooth consistency.

- Nuts with skin, like almonds, can be blended with the skin on. However, for creamier and smoother milk, soak your nuts for 4 hours or until the skin is soft and pops right off. Discard the skins and soaking water, then blend the nuts.

To Make Other Flavors:

Chocolate Milk: Add 1 tablespoon cacao powder.

Strawberry Milk: Add ½ cup strawberries.

Coffee Milk: Replace 1 cup water with 1 cup brewed coffee.

Chocolate Hazelnut Milk: Make a hazelnut milk and add 1 tablespoon cacao powder.

COCONUT MILK

Coconut is a good source of medium-chain triglycerides (MCTs), which are excellent brain fuel. Coconut and MCT oil are excellent for boosting smoothies with another type of good fat.

Total time: 5 minutes • Makes 4 servings

Ingredients:

1 cup coconut flesh or unsweetened shredded coconut

4 cups filtered water

1 seedless date (or 1 tablespoon raw honey or maple syrup)

⅛ teaspoon vanilla extract

Dash of sea salt

Actions:

Put all the ingredients in a high-speed blender, and mix until a smooth consistency is achieved. Drink.

NUT-FREE OAT MILK

Total time: 5 minutes • Makes 4 servings

Ingredients:

1 cup rolled oats

4 cups filtered water

3 seedless dates (or 1 to 2 tablespoons raw honey or maple syrup)

⅛ teaspoon vanilla extract

Dash of sea salt

Actions:

Put all the ingredients in a high-speed blender, and mix until a smooth consistency is achieved. Drink.

Tip:

You can flavor Oat Milk just like Nut Milk and Seed Milk. (See p. 161 for options.)

NUT-FREE TIGERNUT MILK

Tigernut is a root vegetable that makes a delicious, creamy white milk that is absolutely divine! You definitely need a high-speed blender for this one because the tigernuts are a bit hard in texture. But once they are blended, they are an excellent source of vitamins C and E, plus iron, potassium, fiber, and magnesium.

Total time: 5 minutes • Makes 4 servings

Ingredients:

1 cup tigernuts

4 cups filtered water

3 seedless dates (or 1 to 2 tablespoons raw honey or maple syrup)

⅛ teaspoon vanilla extract

Dash of sea salt

Actions:

Put all the ingredients in a high-speed blender, and mix until a smooth consistency is achieved. Drink.

Tip:

You can flavor Tigernut Milk just like Nut Milk and Seed Milk. (See p. 161 for options.)

A Note on Plant-Based Milks

Eliminating dairy is an easy way to avoid a "usual suspect" known to aggravate health conditions, including lung issues, a factor that contributes to anxiety. Nuts, seeds, and oats (common ingredients in plant-based alternatives) are terrific sources of omega-3 fatty acids, which are a top nutrient for brain health.

These nondairy milks take just a few minutes to make. Since they're homemade, they won't have any preservatives or additives like the ones we buy at the store. You can make a big batch of plant-based milk and keep it in a jar in the fridge for up to 14 days.

Drink it on its own as a delicious beverage, add it to your smoothies, and use it to make a breakfast dish or to make your tea and coffee creamier.

BASIC MILKSHAKE FORMULA

This plant-based milkshake can be made with any nondairy milk you like. If you don't have any on hand, you can add all your milk ingredients (following one of the recipes in this chapter) to the blender along with your ice or ice cream!

Total time: 5 minutes • Makes 4 servings

Ingredients:

4 cups nondairy milk (e.g., nut, seed, coconut, oat, or tigernut)

3 cups ice or 1 cup Plant-Based Ice Cream (see p. 254)

Actions:

Put all the ingredients in a blender, mix until a smooth consistency is achieved, and drink.

Variations:

Chocolate Almond Butter Shake: Add 1 tablespoon cacao powder and ¼ cup almond butter.

Chocolate Shake: Add 2 tablespoons cacao powder.

Strawberry Shake: Add 1 cup frozen or fresh strawberries.

Coffee Shake: Replace 1 cup of water with 1 cup brewed coffee.

HOT CHOCOLATE

It is a delicious, soothing, and even romantic act of self-love to enjoy a hot chocolate made from pure cacao. Many studies have shown that cacao immediately relieves stress and anxiety.

Total time: 10 minutes • Makes 1 serving

Ingredients:

1 cup filtered water

1 tablespoon cacao powder

Dash of any type of plant-based milk (nut, seed, or nut-free), to taste

1 tablespoon honey or maple syrup

Actions:

Boil the water in a kettle and pour into a mug. Stir in the rest of the ingredients and enjoy.

Tip:

For a creamy finish, try adding Nut-Free Tigernut Milk or Nut-Free Oat Milk.

Variation:

Spicy Hot Chocolate: Add a dash of cayenne pepper, to taste.

MCT COFFEE LATTE

Dopamine is a neurotransmitter that activates the brain's pleasure centers. Coffee slows down the reabsorption of dopamine, keeping that good feeling going for longer.[7] However, coffee is also a stimulant; the caffeine in it is an antagonist of adenosine, a neurotransmitter that enables us to feel drowsy.[8] Too much coffee makes us jittery.

As long as you don't have more than one a day and take a break from coffee if you feel like you need to, an MCT Coffee Latte will lift your mood.

Total time: 15 minutes • Makes 1 serving

Ingredients:

1½ cups hot coffee

¼ cup plant-based milk of your choice (nut, seed, or nut-free)

1 teaspoon MCT oil

Actions:

1. Brew a cup of coffee with your favorite organic coffee beans.
2. Add the coffee, milk, and oil to a blender and mix for 10 seconds until frothy. Pour into your mug and enjoy!

Variation:

MCT Mocha Latte: Add 1 teaspoon cacao powder.

ANTI-INFLAMMATORY GINGER TEA

This is my classic ginger tea recipe! I recommend that you drink this every night about an hour before bed as a nightcap, as it suppresses sweet cravings and helps drain the lymphatic system, preparing the body for a peaceful, satisfying night's sleep.

You can add all kinds of exciting ingredients to this recipe, like matcha and lemon myrtle leaves, to make interesting therapeutic flavors such as Ginger Lemon Myrtle Tea! I recommend making up a double or triple batch every Sunday, then keeping it in the fridge to drink throughout the week. You can drink it cold or reheat it.

Total time: 10 minutes • Makes 2 servings

Ingredients:

4 cups filtered water

2-inch piece of ginger, diced

Actions:

1. Add water and ginger to a pot and bring to a boil for 5 minutes.

2. Strain the liquid as you pour it into a couple of mugs, then serve.

Tips:

- The water turning slightly yellow/golden is a good sign that the boiling water is extracting the ginger compounds.

- You can also buy ginger tea bags; however, fresh ginger is more potent.

Variations:

Ginger Honey Lemon Tea: Add a squeeze of lemon and 2 teaspoons honey.

Ginger Lavender Tea: Add a serving size of food-grade lavender essential oil.

Ginger Mint Tea: Add a handful of fresh mint leaves.

Ginger Green Tea: Add 1 teaspoon green tea leaves.

Ginger Lemon Myrtle Tea: Add 5 lemon myrtle leaves.

St. John's Wort Ginger Tea: Add 2 drops of St. John's wort liquid extract.

Ginger Rose Tea: Add 1 teaspoon rose hips.

RELAXING BEDTIME TEA

Drink this tea before bed if you would like help having a beautiful, deep, nourishing sleep. The ingredients are all known for inducing sleep. This recipe is very simple to put together, and all these teas are good essentials to have in your pantry for whenever you want a relaxing evening.

Total time: 10 minutes • Makes 1 serving

Ingredients:

2 cups filtered water

1 chamomile tea bag

1 valerian root tea bag

1 passionflower tea bag or liquid extract

1 rose hip tea bag or liquid extract

Actions:

Boil the water in a kettle and pour into a mug. Add in the tea bags and let steep for 5 minutes. (Liquid extracts can be added at the end without steeping.) Enjoy.

LEMON WATER

Total time: 5 minutes • Makes 1 serving

Ingredients:

1 lemon

2 cups filtered water

Actions:

Cut the lemon in half. Squeeze the lemon juice into the water using a citrus press or your hands. Drink.

Tip:

Cut the lemon into quarters if you are squeezing it by hand.

Variation:

Lemon Chlorophyll Water: Add 3 to 18 drops of liquid chlorophyll into your water, depending on your taste and the recommended serving of your brand. (Just a few drops can offer health benefits with no added flavor.)

Lemon Ice Cubes

This recipe is quite profound, although it is so simple. A dear friend came up with this idea as she committed herself to drinking a lemon water every morning upon rising. To save time and avoid procrastination, she simply squeezes lemon juice straight into ice cube trays and keeps it in the freezer at all times. Every morning, she takes out a lemon ice cube and pops it into a cup, adds water, and she is good to go! You can also add a lemon ice cube to your smoothies!

FREEDOM TONIC

A tonic is a restorative beverage that gives us a feeling of vigor and well-being. I call this refreshing drink Freedom Tonic because it provides me with a sense of liberation once I am free of anxiety. It stimulates excitement. The super herbs in this tonic do astonishing things to the body and brain! When I drink this, it puts me in Colorado emotionally; I imagine the days I spent there surrounded by mountains feeling absolutely amazing.

Total time: 10 minutes • Makes 1 serving

Ingredients:

1½ cups sparkling water

½ cup ice

1 handful of fresh mint leaves

½ lime, cut in half

½ teaspoon dried hibiscus flowers

1 drop St. John's wort extract

1 drop rose hip extract

1 drop burdock root

1 drop lavender essential oil (food grade)

1 dropper full of elderberry extract

Actions:

1. Add the sparkling water and ice to a glass. Crush the mint into the water by pressing it down with a spoon.

2. Squeeze the juice of one lime wedge into the water, and then place the other wedge in the glass.

3. Finish by dropping in the hibiscus flowers and extracts. Enjoy this refreshing, tantalizing, and soothing tonic!

Tip:

Substitute 1 drop food-grade essential oil of grapefruit, lime, rosemary, basil, or thyme for the lavender essential oil.

TULSI ELIXIR

Tulsi, also known as holy basil, is an adaptogen, an herb that helps the body adapt to stressors. This particular type of therapeutic elixir is helpful in soothing anxiety because of the herb's immunomodulatory properties. It has been used in the tradition of Ayurveda for millennia.

Total time: 10 minutes • Makes 1 serving

Ingredients:

2 cups boiling filtered water

1 teaspoon dried tulsi (holy basil) leaves

1 teaspoon dried hibiscus flowers

1 teaspoon dried rose petals

1 teaspoon honey

1 drop lavender essential oil (food grade)

1 small lemon wedge

Actions:

1. Add all the ingredients except the lemon to a pot and boil for 5 minutes.

2. Serve in a mug with a squeeze of lemon and enjoy while listening to soothing music.

CHAPTER 8

Easy, Breezy Breakfasts

I recommend you start every day upon rising with a glass of water with lemon juice squeezed into it along with a few drops of chlorophyll. This Lemon Water (p. 168) will be the first thing your cells absorb in the morning when they are most open and hungry for nourishment. That is a powerful way to break the fast!

Next, decide what would be best to eat that day. According to the Mayo Clinic, an ideal breakfast for someone with anxiety is something that includes some protein. "Eating protein at breakfast can help you feel fuller longer and help keep your blood sugar steady so that you have more energy as you start your day."[1]

By contrast, a breakfast consisting of refined carbs and added sugar is destined to create a challenging morning for you because it will induce anxiety and mental instability.

Your breakfast could be a smoothie, a dairy-free milkshake, or a juice—choose any of the recipes in the last chapter. A smoothie is perhaps the best liquid meal replacement, since it can provide 20 to 30 grams of protein and up to 500 calories. All of these beverages are loaded with antioxidants. The recipes in this chapter will be appropriate for mornings when you want to bite into something solid.

In regard to fasting in the morning rather than having breakfast: The way I look at it is that you have to do what is right for you. No two of us are the same. For some people, fasting can cause anxiety—a phenomenon I have talked about previously in this book—and for others, cutting back on calories by going for a longer interval without eating is helpful, as calorie restriction has been said to improve anxiety.[2]

Eating the wrong type of breakfast may be a trigger for anxiety. Processed meat, fried food, refined cereal, and pastries are the absolute worst breakfast foods there are because they are loaded with empty calories. Having them occasionally is not a horrific action. But on a regular basis, they will deplete you. You cannot be the best version of yourself if you are not fueling your body properly.

Whatever you do, do not put white table sugar in your tea or coffee. It's not worth it. Use honey, maple syrup, coconut sugar, monk fruit, or stevia instead. In fact, Vincent M. Pedre, M.D., who prescribes an antianxiety diet to his patients, says, "The spike-and-crash feeling of even a few teaspoons of sugar in your coffee (or any other sugar-filled breakfast) can ramp up anxiety, impair your ability to cope with even the minor stressors life throws your way, and leave you feeling lethargic and groggy." He also recommends starting the day with a smoothie for breakfast, followed by tea and supplements.

It's also a good idea to take your antianxiety supplements in the morning. Some supplements are best taken on an empty stomach; others should be taken during or after a meal for better absorption or to avoid an upset stomach. Check labels for any instructions. I love starting the day with St. John's wort to help me stay feeling sunny and vibrant all day, and kava kava to help me sustain a sense of calm and relaxation throughout the day.

Sample Breakfast Schedule for a Typical Week

You want to rotate your meals a little bit, so you can consume various different nutrients from day to day. In general, for a week of breakfasts, your choices might look like this:

Monday: Smoothie (any kind)

Tuesday: Chia Seed Cereal, Brainiac Porridge, or Granola Cereal

Wednesday: Protein (any kind)

Thursday: Smoothie (any kind)

Friday: Chia Seed Cereal, Brainiac Porridge, or Granola Cereal

Saturday: Protein (any kind)

Sunday: Smoothie (any kind)

Antianxiety Hacks

Here are some antianxiety hacks I suggest as additions to what you're already eating for your first meal of the day, mainly involving small portions of helpful ingredients. For their anti-inflammatory, antioxidant, and neuro-friendly power, try:

- Adding a sprinkle of turmeric to your eggs.
- Drinking ginger, green, or black tea with breakfast.
- Eating an orange or drinking a glass of fresh-squeezed orange juice.
- Eating a handful of cherries, strawberries, or blueberries.
- Consuming cacao in a smoothie, a plant-based milk or milkshake, or in the Genius Chocolate Balls (see p. 246).

CHIA SEED CEREAL

This is a healthier version of a typical breakfast cereal, with the base being chia seeds. Chia is an ancient whole grain that provides a high proportion of alpha-linolenic acid—making it a superb source of plant-based omega-3 fatty acids. Chia seeds contain chlorogenic acid, caffeic acid, myricetin, quercetin, and kaempferol, flavonoids that are believed to be protective of the heart and liver, as well as to provide anticancer and antiaging benefits.[3] Chia is also a great source of dietary fiber, which is beneficial for the digestive system, making you feel full and satiated. Chia seeds have been scientifically established as anti-inflammatory, antidepressant, antianxiety, and immunity-improving. I am excited for you to try chia, an amazing, gluten-free, superior-quality protein!

Fun fact: Chia seeds originated in Mexico and Guatemala and have been part of the human food supply for about 5,500 years. Traditionally, the seeds were used by the Aztec and Mayan peoples in the preparation of their folk medicines, food, and fabric for clothing. In pre-Columbian societies, this crop was second in prominence only to beans.[4]

Total time: 5 minutes • Makes 1 serving

Ingredients:

3 tablespoons chia seeds
½ cup plant-based milk of your choice or filtered water

Toppings (of your choosing):

Blueberries
Flax meal
Hempseeds

Organic SunButter
Roasted walnuts
Strawberries

Actions:

1. Place the chia seeds and liquid into a cereal bowl. Soak for 10 minutes.
2. Add the toppings and eat.

Tip:

For sweeter cereal, add 1 teaspoon raw honey, maple syrup, or chopped dates.

Variations:

Chia Hempseed Cereal: Add 1 tablespoon hempseeds.

Oatmeal Chia Seed Cereal: Add 1 tablespoon whole rolled oats.

BRAINIAC PORRIDGE

Porridge, by tradition, is a bowl of boiled crushed or ground grains served as breakfast cereal. Heated oats or oatmeal is perhaps the most recognizable type of porridge. This breakfast gives me a warm and fuzzy feeling inside. For so many years, I avoided oats because I thought they were too "carby," and grains had gotten such a bad rap in the media; however, in doing my research for this book I discovered so many health benefits of oats that I started to incorporate them in my diet again—and I am so glad I did. Oats are said to significantly increase healthy brain activity, which is why I named this "Brainiac" Porridge.

Total time: 5 minutes • Makes 1 serving

Ingredients:

For the porridge:

⅓ cup organic rolled oats   ⅔ cup plant-based milk

Toppings (of your choosing):

Almond butter	Honey
Almonds	Macadamia nuts
Apples	Nectarines
Apricots	Nutiva Coconut Manna
Bananas	Organic SunButter
Blueberries	Peaches
Brazil nuts	Pecans
Cacao nibs	Pomegranates
Chia seeds	Pumpkin seeds
Cinnamon	Rose petals
Coconut sugar	Sunflower seeds
Flax meal	Walnuts

Actions:

1. Add the oats and milk to a pot and bring to a boil. Allow the mixture to boil for a few minutes until the oats are cooked to your liking.

2. Serve the porridge in a bowl with the toppings of your choice. Get creative and make some food art!

Tip:

Add 1 tablespoon MCT oil to your porridge as a brain booster.

OVERNIGHT OATS WITH CHOCOLATE AVOCADO MOUSSE

Prepping your breakfast tonight will make for a smoother morning tomorrow. With just a few minutes and a handful of ingredients, you can have delicious breakfast oats waiting for you in the refrigerator to eat at home or grab and go.

Total time: 5 minutes • Makes 2 servings

Ingredients:

1 cup oats

1 tablespoon chia seeds

1 cup plant-based milk (nut, seed, or other)

Chocolate Avocado Mousse (see p. 249)

Actions:

1. Divide the oats, chia seeds, and plant milk into 2 jars. Refrigerate overnight to set.

2. Make the Chocolate Avocado Mousse and serve on top of the oats.

3. Serve with fresh fruit, nuts, and/or granola.

GRANOLA CEREAL

This recipe makes a great breakfast cereal. Just add some milk and your choice of toppings and it can fulfill your wildest cereal craving. Make an extra batch and store in a glass jar so you always have granola on hand as a snack.

Total time: 20 minutes • Makes 4 servings

Ingredients:

1½ cups almond butter or organic SunButter

1 cup oats

½ cup tigernut flour or almond flour

2 tablespoons honey

⅓ cup walnuts, chopped

5 dates, seeded

¼ cup chia seeds

¼ cup hempseeds

1 tablespoon coconut oil

1 tablespoon MCT oil

¼ teaspoon vanilla extract

¼ teaspoon sea salt

4 cups plant-based milk (nut, seed, or other)

Toppings:

Fresh or dried fruits of your choice: blueberries or chopped/sliced apples, apricots, and bananas, for instance

Actions:

1. Preheat the oven to 325°F.

2. Mix all the ingredients in a bowl until they are moist enough to stick together.

3. Place the mixture on a baking tray in clumps and bake for 9 minutes, or until just golden.

4. Assemble: Add 1 cup plant-based milk to each bowl, then add the baked granola, then the toppings.

SUNBUTTER PROTEIN GRANOLA BARS

These bars make an excellent grab-and-go breakfast, or even a snack any time of day.

Total time: 8 minutes • Makes 21 bars

Ingredients:

Coconut oil, for greasing the baking dish

1½ cups organic SunButter

1 cup oats

½ cup tigernut flour

½ cup almond flour

2 tablespoons honey

2 tablespoons MCT oil

2 seedless dates

1 teaspoon maca powder

¼ cup chia seeds

¼ cup hempseeds

1 scoop Nutiva vanilla-flavored plant protein

Actions:

1. Grease a 9 x 13-inch glass baking dish with coconut oil.

2. Mix all the other ingredients in a bowl until they are moist enough to stick together. If the mixture is too dry to mold, add a bit of filtered water.

3. Pat the mixture into the greased dish. You can bake the mixture for 9 minutes at 325°F or keep it raw. Cut it into squares before serving.

Tip:

For an antioxidant boost, add ½ teaspoon of spirulina powder.

BRAIN BOWL

The Brain Bowl is a smoothie bowl that uses spirulina or Blue Majik, a product that is a blend of spirulina and other algae powders. If you use the latter, the bowl will be a gorgeous bright blue! The bright blue looks like a fake color from food coloring, but it's really natural—coming from C-phycocyanin, a type of storage protein sourced from seeds that is rich in amino acids. You will be happy just looking at it, and bonus: It makes a gorgeous photo.

A smoothie bowl is just as it sounds, a smoothie in a bowl. It's made this way so you can add toppings like fresh blueberries, strawberries, and cacao nibs artfully and enjoy it at breakfast, or for any meal for that matter. It's a delightful antioxidant treat.

Total time: 10 minutes • Makes 1 serving

Ingredients:

For the base:

1 frozen banana

½ cup frozen blueberries

1 cup coconut milk

½ kiwifruit

½ teaspoon spirulina powder or Blue Majik

1 teaspoon hempseeds

Toppings:

½ kiwifruit, sliced

2 tablespoons walnuts

1 teaspoon chia seeds

½ teaspoon flax meal or seeds

1 tablespoon blueberries

1 tablespoon blackberries

2 strawberries, sliced

1 teaspoon cacao nibs

Actions:

1. Blend all the ingredients for the base in a blender until smooth.

2. Pour the smoothie into a bowl and add the toppings.

AÇAI BOWL

Açai is incredibly high in antioxidants, which neutralize that anxiety-causing oxidative stress. The cool thing about this smoothie bowl is its versatility: You can eat it for breakfast, lunch, or dinner, or as a snack or dessert! It's topped with delicious blueberries, strawberries, and cacao nibs.

Total time: 6 minutes • Makes 1 serving

Ingredients:

For the base:

2 Sambazon Açaí Superfruit Packs

1 frozen banana

¼ cup plant-based milk of your choice

Toppings:

1 teaspoon cacao nibs

4 strawberries, sliced

2 tablespoons blueberries

1 to 2 tablespoons granola

Actions:

1. Blend all the ingredients for the base in a blender until smooth.

2. Pour the smoothie into a bowl and add the toppings.

Variation:

Chocolate Açai Bowl: Add 2 teaspoons cacao powder to the base mixture before blending.

BLUEBERRY MUFFINS

Total time: 50 minutes • Makes 12 muffins

Ingredients:

2 tablespoons flax meal

2 tablespoons filtered water

½ cup almond milk

1 teaspoon apple cider vinegar

1½ teaspoons baking soda

2 organic apples or ½ cup applesauce

1 tablespoon MCT oil

¼ cup coconut oil

⅓ cup maple syrup

¼ cup coconut sugar

½ teaspoon sea salt

1 cup organic blueberries

2 tablespoons chia seeds

For the gluten-free flour mix:

1 tablespoon potato starch

2 tablespoons tapioca flour

¼ cup tigernut flour

1 tablespoon brown rice flour

¾ cup Nutiva plant-based protein powder

¼ cup almond flour

Actions:

1. Preheat the oven to 375°F and line a 12-cup muffin tray with paper baking cups.

2. Make an egg replacement: Mix the flax and water together in a small cup until well combined. Let the mixture sit for 10 minutes until it becomes gummy like eggs. Set aside.

3. Combine all the ingredients of the gluten-free flour mix in a separate bowl and set aside.

4. Mix the almond milk, apple cider vinegar, and baking soda in a separate bowl until well combined. Set aside.

5. Peel and core the apples. Mix in a blender or food processor with the MCT oil until you have an applesauce.

6. Mix the coconut oil, maple syrup, coconut sugar, and applesauce in a separate large bowl. Add the egg replacement (see step 2) to the mixture in this bowl and whisk.

7. Add the almond milk mixture and stir well.

8. Add the sea salt and gluten-free flour mix, and stir well.

9. Gently stir in the blueberries and chia seeds.

10. Pour the batter evenly among 12 baking cups and bake for 24 minutes, or until golden brown. When you poke the center of a muffin with a toothpick, it should come out dry.

11. Let the muffins cool for 15 minutes, then dig in and enjoy.

BASIC OMELET FORMULA

Eggs are a protein-rich breakfast! And please eat the entire egg: There are benefits in eating both the egg whites, which contain tryptophan—a precursor to serotonin—and the egg yolks, which contain vitamins A, D, E, and K along with omega-3 fats.

An omelet is delicious, quick, and high in protein. With vegetables added, it also provides the body with high amounts of antioxidants. Omelets make great breakfasts, lunches, and dinners.

The basic concept of an omelet is heating up some oil in a pan, whisking the egg with the spices of your choice in a bowl, then pouring the batter into the hot pan. When the top surface has thickened and no visible egg or moisture remains, you put toppings of your choice on one half of the omelet, then fold the other half over and cook until it's done. You can use plain eggs or add 1 tablespoon milk or filtered water per egg to the mixture.

Total time: 10 minutes • Makes 2 servings

Ingredients:

1 tablespoon oil, for cooking (see options below)

4 large eggs

1 tablespoon plant milk or water

Black pepper and sea salt, to taste

Toppings (see suggestions below)

Choose your oil:

Extra-virgin coconut oil

Extra-virgin olive oil

Avocado oil

Choose your toppings:

Nutritional yeast, as a cheese alternative

Organic cheese, shreds or thin slices

Artichoke, chopped

Avocado, sliced

Basil, chopped or powder

Cayenne pepper

Cilantro, chopped or powder

Cumin powder

Scallions

Kale, chopped

Organic turkey, chopped

Parsley, chopped

Spinach, chopped

Tomatoes, chopped

Turmeric

Zucchini, chopped

Actions:

1. Heat the oil in a frying pan over medium heat. Crack the eggs into a bowl, add milk or water and seasonings, then whisk with a fork. Pour the mixture into the pan.

2. Cook until the top of the egg mixture begins to firm, then add your toppings on half the surface. Fold the other half over using a spatula and continue cooking for 30 to 60 seconds.

3. Flip the omelet over with a spatula, then continue cooking until desired doneness is achieved. Invert the pan to release the omelet or slide it onto plates and serve immediately. Enjoy!

TURKEY OMELET

Start your day with a savory serving of tryptophan.

Ingredients:

1 tablespoon extra-virgin coconut oil

4 large eggs

1 tablespoon fresh parsley, chopped

¼ teaspoon onion powder

½ teaspoon garlic, minced

4 slices turkey, chopped

½ small tomato, sliced

MEDITERRANEAN OMELET

The eating habits of people from the Mediterranean region have been proven by many studies to have a multitude of health benefits, including alleviating symptoms of depression and anxiety, and even reducing one's risk of cancer.

Ingredients:

1 tablespoon extra-virgin olive oil

4 large eggs

2 tablespoons sliced olives

½ cup spinach

½ small tomato, sliced

1 tablespoon fresh parsley, chopped

½ teaspoon garlic, minced

2 tablespoons organic cheese or 1 tablespoon nutritional yeast

HASH BROWNS

The ultimate comfort food! Grate up a bunch of potatoes for hash browns and keep these in an airtight container in your freezer so you can have a fun, delicious, and vitamin C–rich snack, breakfast, lunch, or dinner anytime! Fast-food fried potatoes will cause anxiety, but homemade potato recipes like this one, made with organic potatoes, will help reduce anxiety.

Potatoes are an amazing root vegetable. Aboriginal people from the area where I grew up in Australia say they are "grounding" because they are a root. (The same concept can be applied as to why ginger, carrots, and turmeric are good for us.)

The modern science community has proven potatoes to be a healthy, functional food—when eaten in the right way, of course. Obviously, a fast-food restaurant that serves fried potatoes is probably not making them in the most healthful manner, and greasy fast-food fries will cause damage to our health. By comparison, organic potatoes grown in nutrient-rich soil and cooked in coconut oil or extra-virgin olive oil, or baked, provide us with a lot of health benefits, including the reduction of anxiety.

Unfortunately, a couple of decades ago, the white potato was labeled as a "food to avoid" because of inconsistent epidemiologic research showing that a Western dietary pattern was linked to weight gain and increased risk of type 2 diabetes. The trouble with the research was that it included all white potatoes regardless of their preparation method.

Today we know better. White potatoes prepared in the right ways are healthful and continue to be a staple food in my diet. They play an important role in our vegetable intake, as they are a low-cost source of critical nutrients, which include potassium, magnesium, dietary fiber, resistant starch, vitamin B_6, and vitamin C, as well as high-quality protein and satiating carbohydrates.[5] Potatoes exceed the recommended levels for four of the nine essential amino acids—lysine, methionine, threonine, and tryptophan—demonstrating that potato protein is of high quality.[6]

If you've been avoiding potatoes, these delectable hash browns are your chance to bring them back!

Total time: 10 minutes • Makes 1 to 2 servings

Ingredients:

1 tablespoon coconut oil or avocado oil, for cooking

1 large organic potato

Dash of turmeric

Dash of rosemary

Dash of sea salt

Dash of black pepper

Actions:

1. Heat a frying pan with the oil over medium heat. Meanwhile, peel and grate the potato into a bowl. Add the turmeric and rosemary and mix well.

2. Stir-fry the potato for 8 minutes, or until cooked to your liking.

3. Season with sea salt and black pepper.

CHAPTER 9

Plant-Based Energizing Lunches and Healing Dinners

Here you can find lunch and dinner dishes that are plant-based and entirely vegan. They are all gluten-free and high in antioxidants. Consuming these dishes is a wonderful way to put some more tasty plant foods into your diet. The beauty is that every type of eater can enjoy these, even omnivorous fish and meat eaters.

WALNUT "MEATBALLS" WITH ZOODLES

Walnut "meatballs" go well on a bed of zucchini noodles—aka zoodles—for a completely raw dish. For a meal with both raw and cooked components, you can substitute gluten-free pasta (such as chickpea or bean pasta) for the zoodles. These hybrid dishes offer the best of both worlds: the health benefits of raw foods and the comfort of a home-cooked meal!

Total time: 10 minutes • Makes 12 1-inch balls (4 servings)

Ingredients:

For the "meatballs":

1½ cups walnuts

1 cup sun-dried tomatoes

2 tablespoons extra-virgin olive oil

1 teaspoon organic SunButter

1 teaspoon dried sage

1 teaspoon fennel seeds

1 teaspoon dried thyme

1 teaspoon dried rosemary

1 teaspoon dried oregano

Pinch of black pepper

Pinch of cayenne pepper

Pinch of sea salt

For the zoodles:

4 small zucchinis, peeled

Actions:

1. Add all the "meatball" ingredients to your blender and mix for 5 minutes, or until well combined. The mixture should be moist and stick together. Roll the mixture with your hands to make about 12 one-inch balls.

2. Make the zoodles by adding the zucchini to a pasta spiralizer or simply use a vegetable peeler to make thin noodle shapes.

3. Divide the pasta and "meatballs" onto 4 plates and serve.

Tips:

- Skip the noodles! Wrap up a few of the walnut balls in lettuce, along with your desired toppings, to make raw tacos.

- If you do not have a blender, use a mortar and pestle to crush the walnuts. Then dice the sun-dried tomatoes and mix everything together in a bowl.

- For a nut-free version, use pumpkin seeds, hempseeds, or sunflower seeds instead of walnuts.

- You can use food-grade essential oils instead of dried herbs, but be sparing. Start with just the amount of oil you get when you dip a clean toothpick in the bottle, then increase the quantity, to taste. Essential oils are concentrated, and their intensity varies from oil to oil. Most times only a drop or two is needed to substitute for dried herbs. Definitely use only a toothpickful if adding oregano essential oil, as the flavor is quite strong.

CHICKPEA BURGERS

Could chickpeas be the next new superfood? Emerging research suggests that chickpeas play a beneficial role in weight management as well as glucose and insulin regulation. They also have a positive impact on some markers of cardiovascular disease. Raw or cooked chickpeas contain dietary bioactive compounds such as phytic acid, sterols, tannins, carotenoids, and other polyphenols such as isoflavones, whose benefits may extend beyond our basic nutritional requirements.

Total time: 10 minutes • Makes 4 burgers

Ingredients:

2 tablespoons extra-virgin coconut oil, for cooking

One 14-ounce can chickpeas, drained

3 tablespoons almond flour or tigernut flour

1 tablespoon tapioca flour

1 tablespoon flax meal

2 teaspoons crushed garlic

1 teaspoon sea salt

1 teaspoon onion powder

¼ teaspoon cumin seeds

½ teaspoon cumin powder

¼ teaspoon turmeric

¼ teaspoon fennel

¼ teaspoon sage

¼ teaspoon rosemary

⅛ teaspoon oregano

Actions:

1. Heat the oil in a large pan over medium heat. Mash the chickpeas, then combine with the rest of the ingredients. Taste the mixture and add more spices or salt to your liking.

2. Divide the mixture into 4 equal parts and shape into patties.

3. Fry the patties until golden, about 4 minutes on each side.

Variation:

Bean Burgers: Substitute black beans for the chickpeas.

BROCCOLI POPCORN

Try this delicious take on a healthy popcorn, made with a twist!

Total time: 10 minutes • Makes 4 servings

Ingredients:

2½ tablespoons extra-virgin olive oil or coconut oil

½ cup nutritional yeast

¾ teaspoon sea salt

1 head of broccoli, chopped into bite-size pieces

Actions:

1. Preheat the oven to 325°F.

2. Mix the oil, nutritional yeast, and salt in a large bowl until combined. Add the broccoli to the mixture and toss until the pieces are well coated.

3. Place the broccoli on a baking tray and bake for 20 minutes, or until just golden brown.

Tips:

*   For extra flavor, add 1 tablespoon sesame seeds.

*   For extra flavor and protein, add 1 tablespoon organic SunButter.

*   Use butter-flavored Nutiva Coconut Oil for that "movie popcorn" flavor.

Variation:

Cauliflower Popcorn: Substitute an equal amount of cauliflower for the broccoli.

CREAMY, DELICIOUS VEGAN GF MAC 'N' CHEESE

It took me years to finally tweak this recipe to perfection! It is creamy, so smooth, absolutely delicious, and healthy! Also, it's dairy-free and gluten-free, made using whole-food ingredients for a hearty, nutrient-rich mac 'n' cheese.

Total time: 20 minutes • Makes 4 servings

Ingredients:

1 box Explore Cuisine Chickpea Fusilli

¼ cup butter-flavored Nutiva Coconut Oil

2 garlic cloves, minced

¼ cup tapioca flour

2 cups almond milk or other nut milk

¼ cup nutritional yeast

3 tablespoons Raw "Parmesan" Cheese (see p. 223) or store-bought vegan cheese, optional

½ teaspoon sea salt

¼ teaspoon thyme

¼ teaspoon rosemary

¼ teaspoon black pepper

Actions:

1. Cook the pasta as per packet directions. Drain and set aside.

2. While the pasta is cooking, heat the oil over medium heat in a medium cooking pot. Add the garlic, and cook for 2 minutes until just golden. Add in the tapioca flour and saute for 1 minute.

3. Slowly add in the almond milk while whisking, continuing to cook over medium heat for 2 minutes.

4. Whisk in the nutritional yeast and vegan cheese, if using. The sauce will be a little clumpy at first, so keep stirring in the milk until it's completely smooth. You can also use a hand blender or transfer the mixture to a blender if you want a smoother consistency.

5. Add the pasta to the pot of hot sauce and mix well with the seasonings, then serve in bowls.

Tips:

- Serve with any toppings you like. I love adding organic peas, corn, chopped fresh parsley, and dried chili pepper to mine.

- If you intend to use Raw "Parmesan" Cheese, then you will have to prepare it a day ahead since it takes 12 hours to make in a dehydrator. Store-bought is a convenience.

PASTA PRIMAVERA

This colorful dish literally bounces in your mouth! It's a great combo of a nutrient-dense pasta—choose from brown rice, lentil, or chickpea pasta—and a vibrant array of antioxidant vegetables. Packed with protein and nutrient-richness, it's bound to leave you feeling vibrantly healthy.

Total time: 30 minutes • Makes 4 servings

Ingredients:

2 cups uncooked gluten-free pasta (brown rice, lentil, or chickpea)

¼ cup extra-virgin coconut oil

1 yellow onion, chopped

2 garlic cloves, diced

1 head of broccoli, including stems, chopped into bite-size pieces (2 to 3 cups)

1 cup spinach

1 cup fresh or frozen peas

2 carrots, chopped in thick slices

1 cup broccoli sprouts

Sea salt and cracked black pepper, to taste

Actions:

1. Place the pasta in a large pot and cook as per box instructions. Drain and set aside.

2. While the pasta is cooking, heat the coconut oil in a frying pan over medium heat. Add the onion and garlic and fry, stirring frequently, until the vegetables turn golden brown.

3. Add the broccoli to the frying pan. Continue frying, stirring frequently, until the broccoli is just tender.

4. Add the cooked pasta to the pan with the vegetables and toss to combine. Immediately after, add the spinach, peas, carrots, and broccoli sprouts and toss for a few minutes, until the flavors and oils are combined.

5. Season with sea salt and pepper, to taste.

Tips:

- Feel free to add other vegetables to this dish, especially green ones!

- Add some honey to make it nice and sweet.

- Add some other seasonings if you wish, like turmeric and sesame seeds.

BRAIN BOWL WITH WALNUT PESTO SAUCE

A hearty bowl with different textures and flavors to satisfy every taste, made with brain-nourishing ingredients. There is such variety in this bowl that it is sure to hit the spot.

Total time: 40 minutes • Makes 2 servings

Ingredients:

½ cup quinoa

½ cup lentils

1 tablespoon extra-virgin coconut oil

1 large carrot, cubed

1 teaspoon ginger, diced

1 tablespoon honey

For the Walnut Pesto Sauce:

1 cup fresh basil

¼ cup broccoli sprouts

Juice of 1 lemon

1 garlic clove

½ teaspoon sea salt

1 cup spinach

2 cups raw walnuts

⅓ cup extra-virgin olive oil

½ cup pinto beans (or beans of your choice)

1 avocado, chopped in half and then sliced

¼ cup kimchi or sauerkraut

Fresh cilantro

Fresh parsley

⅓ cup broccoli sprouts

Dash of cayenne pepper or chili flakes, optional

Toppings:

Actions:

1. Bring a pot of water to a boil, and add the quinoa and lentils. Cook until the lentils are done, about 20 minutes, then drain.

2. Meanwhile, add the coconut oil to a frying pan with the carrot and ginger. Stir-fry at medium-high heat for a few minutes, and then add the honey. Let the mixture cook until the carrot is softened.

3. Make the Walnut Pesto Sauce by adding all the ingredients to a blender and mixing until almost smooth (some chunks are nice).

4. Transfer the lentils and quinoa to 2 bowls, then add the toppings. Enjoy!

Tip:

To save time on cooking the quinoa and lentils, you can use Explore Cuisine Green Lentil Penne instead, which cooks in 10 minutes.

TURMERIC CAULIFLOWER RICE

One way to spice up a side dish like rice is by adding some turmeric along with ginger, garlic, and black pepper. This makes for a delicious and comforting meal or side dish. Here we use cauliflower instead of rice, so it's grain-free.

Total time: 45 minutes • Makes 4 servings

Ingredients:

1 head of cauliflower

2 tablespoons extra-virgin coconut oil

1 yellow onion, chopped

2 tablespoons chopped garlic

1 tablespoon chopped ginger

2 tablespoons turmeric powder

½ teaspoon black pepper

1 carrot, cut into finely sliced rounds

Actions:

1. Separate the cauliflower into chunks to fit into your food processor, then process into pieces the size of rice. Don't blend too far or you could end up with cauliflower soup.

2. Heat the coconut oil in a frying pan over medium heat. Add the onion, garlic, ginger, turmeric, black pepper, and carrots and fry the mixture until the vegetables are just tender.

3. Add the cauliflower rice to the carrot mixture in the pan and stir-fry for 7 to 10 minutes, until the vegetables are soft and ready to eat!

RAINBOW VEGGIE STIR-FRY

Who said veggie stir-fries are boring? Not with this rainbow assortment of vegetables and freshly squeezed orange juice.

Total time: 35 minutes • Makes 4 servings

Ingredients:

¼ cup extra-virgin coconut oil

1 small yellow onion, chopped

4 large garlic cloves, chopped

1-inch piece of ginger, chopped

1 teaspoon turmeric powder

1 teaspoon cumin

1 teaspoon thyme

½ teaspoon sea salt

4 brussels sprouts, chopped

1 large carrot, chopped

½ head of broccoli, chopped

1 cup chopped bok choy

½ head of cauliflower, chopped

¼ small beet, cut into cubes

1 cup spinach

1 cup green beans

Juice from 2 oranges

1 teaspoon sesame seeds

½ cup broccoli sprouts

Actions:

1. Heat the oil in a wok or frying pan, then add the onion and garlic. Sauté for 2 minutes, then add the ginger. Sauté for another minute, then add the turmeric, cumin, thyme, and sea salt.

2. Add the vegetables to the onion mixture and stir-fry until they become tender, about 10 to 15 minutes. Add the orange juice (hand squeezed is okay).

3. Sprinkle the sesame seeds and broccoli sprouts over each serving, along with salt and pepper to taste.

Tip:

Serve over quinoa.

STIR-FRIED SATAY NOODLES

Stay in and make this Asian-inspired recipe.

Total time: 30 minutes • Makes 4 servings

Ingredients:

For the sauce:

3 tablespoons butter-flavored Nutiva Coconut Oil

2 scallions, chopped

1 tablespoon crushed garlic

1 tablespoon diced fresh ginger

⅓ cup organic SunButter

2 tablespoons hot sauce

1 tablespoon apple cider vinegar

3 tablespoons maple syrup

¼ teaspoon turmeric

¼ teaspoon sea salt

2 tablespoons lime juice

½ teaspoon dried cilantro

⅓ cup Bragg Liquid Aminos

½ teaspoon red chili flakes, optional

1 tablespoon MCT oil

For the stir-fry:

2 tablespoons sesame seed oil

1 teaspoon crushed garlic

2 scallions, chopped

1 small head of broccoli, chopped into bite-size pieces

1 large carrot, cut into strips

1 red pepper, cut into strips

Any other vegetables you like— sliced into strips!

For the pasta:

1 box Explore Cuisine Chickpea Spaghetti

Fresh cilantro, for garnish

Actions:

1. Make the satay sauce first. Heat the coconut oil in a saucepan over medium heat with the scallions, garlic, and ginger. Sauté until golden brown, about 4 minutes. Reduce the heat to low and add in the remaining sauce ingredients. Continue to cook, stirring constantly, for 7 minutes, or until the sauce thickens. Set aside.

2. Make the stir-fry by adding the sesame seed oil, garlic, and scallions, to a large, hot frying pan. Stir-fry over medium heat for a couple minutes, then add the vegetables and cook until they are tender.

3. Pour the satay sauce over the vegetables in the pan and mix well. Set aside.

4. Cook the pasta per the box instructions. Drain and add to the vegetable satay stir-fry and toss until well combined. Serve garnished with fresh cilantro.

CAULIFLOWER-CHEESE PESTO LASAGNA

This is gluten-free and dairy-free as well as vegan. It's made with no-boil green lentil lasagna sheets, which are layered with two distinct and delicious homemade sauces for a comforting dish that's full of Italian-inspired taste. Made with better-for-you ingredients, the pesto gives the meal a bright-tasting quality from the basil and the spinach, offering extra health benefits. The cauliflower-based Alfredo sauce really completes this satisfying lunch or dinner.

When cooking, make sure to use plenty of sauce so the lasagna sheets soak up the flavor—that is the key to using no-boil noodles. You can also enjoy the leftovers the next day. Make some for dinner today and enjoy the rest for lunch tomorrow.

Total time: 1 hour • Makes 4 servings

Ingredients:

For the pesto:

1 cup fresh basil leaves

½ cup spinach

2 garlic cloves, peeled

3 tablespoons pine nuts

⅓ cup nutritional yeast

⅓ cup extra-virgin olive oil

¼ teaspoon sea salt

For the Alfredo sauce:

1 tablespoon butter-flavored Nutiva Coconut Oil

2 teaspoons crushed garlic

1 shallot, thinly sliced

1 cup cashew milk or other nut milk

2 cups vegetable broth

3 cups cauliflower florets

¼ cup nutritional yeast

1 tablespoon lemon juice

1 tablespoon extra-virgin olive oil

¼ teaspoon dried thyme

¼ teaspoon dried oregano

¼ teaspoon sea salt

¼ teaspoon black pepper

For the lasagna:

1 pack Explore Cuisine Green Lentil Lasagna

1 tablespoon nutritional yeast

1 tablespoon pine nuts

Actions:

Preheat the oven to 375°F.

1. *For the pesto:* Pulse the ingredients in a food processor until well combined. Set aside.

2. *For the Alfredo sauce:* Sauté the coconut oil, garlic, and shallot in a medium saucepan over medium heat until fragrant and golden.

3. Stir in the milk and vegetable broth. Increase the heat and bring the mixture to a medium boil.

4. Add the cauliflower florets to the saucepan. Lower the heat to medium, cover, and cook for 10 minutes, or until the cauliflower is soft.

5. Combine the cauliflower mixture and the remaining Alfredo sauce ingredients in a blender and blend on high until creamy and smooth.

6. *To assemble the lasagna:* Spread a layer of Alfredo sauce in a square (9 x 9-inch) or rectangular (9 x 13-inch) baking dish. Layer 4 lasagna sheets over the sauce. Spread a layer of pesto sauce over the lasagna, then add another layer of 4 lasagna sheets. Alternate layering the Alfredo sauce, 4 sheets of pasta, pesto, and 4 sheets of pasta until all the sheets are used, reserving enough pesto for the top layer. Note: Depending on the size of the dish, you may be preparing 3 or 4 layers.

7. Sprinkle the nutritional yeast and pine nuts over the top pesto layer.

8. Bake the lasagna in the oven for 40 minutes, until the noodles are cooked through.

CAULIFLOWER CHEESE FRIES

This recipe is a fun, dairy-free twist on cheese fries. Thick, creamy, smooth, and delicious. Wow, what a combo! These fries are made in the oven and come out nice and golden and crispy, because after the potato is cut, it is coated with potato starch before cooking. We're aiming for the fries to be crunchy on the outside and soft in the inside.

Total time: 40 minutes • Makes 4 servings

Ingredients:

For the fries:

1 tablespoon sea salt

4 large organic potatoes (white potatoes or sweet potatoes)

1 teaspoon chopped garlic

1 tablespoon extra-virgin olive oil

2 tablespoons potato starch

For the cauliflower cheese:

3 cups chopped cauliflower (from 1 small head of cauliflower)

1 cup plant-based milk of your choice

¼ cup nutritional yeast

1 tablespoon lemon juice (from about ½ lemon)

1 tablespoon extra-virgin olive oil

¼ teaspoon dried thyme

½ teaspoon sea salt

¼ teaspoon black pepper

¼ teaspoon dried rosemary

½ teaspoon tapioca flour

¼ teaspoon potato starch

½ teaspoon garlic salt

Actions:

1. Preheat the oven to 450°F.

2. Bring a pot of water to a boil with a tablespoon of sea salt.

3. While the water is boiling, prepare the fries: Cut the potatoes into the shape of thick fries. Add the potatoes to the boiling water and reduce the heat to low. Simmer for about 10 minutes, until soft. Poke a potato with a knife to see if it is partially cooked—it shouldn't be cooked all the way through yet.

4. Drain the potatoes and place them on a baking tray, then coat them well with garlic and extra-virgin olive oil. Next, sprinkle the potato starch over the potatoes, pressing the fries into the starch so they are evenly covered. Make sure there are no chunks of potato starch on the fries.

5. Bake for 10 to 15 minutes, until the potatoes are golden brown.

6. While the potatoes are bubbling away, make the cauliflower cheese: Bring a small saucepan of water to a boil. Add the cauliflower florets and cook for 10 to 15 minutes, or until the cauliflower is soft. Drain.

7. Transfer the cauliflower to a blender along with the rest of the cauliflower cheese ingredients. Blend on high until the mixture is creamy and smooth. Return the cauliflower cheese mixture to the empty saucepan (no water), and simmer over low heat to keep it warm until the potatoes are cooked.

8. Pour the cauliflower cheese over the fries, serve, and enjoy!

CHAPTER 10

Sensational Soups, Super Salads, and Delicious Dressings

Consuming soups and salads, along with the right dressings, is a way to know for sure that you are doing something really healthy for your body. All of the soups, salads, and dressings in this chapter are gluten-free, dairy-free, and refined sugar–free. There are a variety of vegan recipes as well as some that include chicken.

If you want to add protein to a vegan soup or salad, you can add fish or meat. For example, you could make an animal protein such as the Walnut-Crusted Chicken, and add it to any salad recipe. I recommend making extra chicken for dinner one night, and reserving some for your salad the next day.

Soups are so soothing when we're feeling anxious. They warm the body as they boost the immune system. I recommend making an extra-big batch of soup, and then freezing some so you can heat it up in a pot when you need a quick meal on a busy day. Also, if an anxiety attack hits, rather than having to scramble around to make a decision on what food to eat, if you have a ready-made soup in the freezer, you can relax. Knowing that lunch or dinner is already taken care of can be a good way to soothe those nerves.

Avocado slices, broccoli sprouts, and fresh herbs like parsley and cilantro make excellent soup toppings. And because we are focusing on brain-boosting ingredients, remember that you can add a bit of extra-virgin olive oil and MCT oil to every soup.

I've got another labor-saving idea for you. All of these salads can be made as a mason jar salad! This technique is life-changing, especially for a busy mom or an active person. You can make up to seven days' worth of salads, store them in mason jars, and then take one to work with you, or just pull it from the fridge at home and tip it all out into a bowl. Toss with dressing. Salad stays fresh longer when stored in a jar!

CHICKEN NOODLE SOUP

Chicken can have a positive effect on your feelings of stress as it contains the amino acid tryptophan, which we know helps the brain produce feel-good chemicals. Chicken Noodle Soup for the soul is right! And this recipe is made with wholesome vegetables and a lovely, soft, gluten-free noodle.

Total time: 35 minutes • Makes 4 servings

Ingredients:

1 tablespoon coconut oil

2 celery stalks, chopped

1 large carrot, chopped

1 yellow onion, sliced

2 garlic cloves, minced

½ teaspoon dried basil

½ teaspoon dried oregano

½ teaspoon dried thyme

¼ teaspoon sea salt

¼ teaspoon pepper

56 ounces chicken broth

14 ounces vegetable broth

½ pound organic chicken, cut into thin strips

Your choice of noodles: Explore Cuisine gluten-free rice noodles, like the Organic Brown Rice Ramen Noodles, or Chickpea Spaghetti

Broccoli sprouts, for serving

Actions:

1. Place the oil, celery, carrot, onion, and garlic in a large pot and cook for 1 minute over medium-high heat, stirring. Add the remaining ingredients, except for the noodles and sprouts.

2. Bring to a boil and allow to cook for 7 minutes.

3. Add the noodles and cook until they are done according to the package instructions. The soup is ready when the chicken is cooked through (no pinkness at the center) and the noodles are done.

4. Serve topped with broccoli sprouts.

Variation:

Veggie Noodle Soup: You can make this entirely plant-based by using 70 ounces of vegetable broth and no chicken.

IMMUNE-BOOSTING VEGETABLE SOUP

This is the recipe for those days when you want to boost your immune system and feel uplifted and comforted.

Total time: 40 minutes • Makes 4 servings

Ingredients:

5 cups filtered water

1 yellow onion, sliced

4 garlic cloves, chopped

½ teaspoon dried thyme or 1 tablespoon fresh thyme

½ teaspoon dried parsley or 1 tablespoon fresh parsley

½ teaspoon dried oregano

1 teaspoon sea salt

¼ teaspoon black pepper

½ head of cauliflower, chopped

½ head of broccoli, chopped

1 large carrot, chopped

2 large potatoes, chopped into cubes

2 celery stalks, chopped

2 large tomatoes, chopped into cubes

2 tablespoons extra-virgin olive oil

2 tablespoons MCT oil

Dash of cayenne pepper, optional

Actions:

1. Place the water, onion, garlic, herbs, and spices in a large pot over high heat and bring to a boil. Meanwhile, chop the vegetables.

2. Add the vegetables and oils to the pot and allow the mixture to boil for another 15 minutes, until the vegetables are softer.

Tip:

To bump up the protein in this soup, you could add beans (vegan option), Walnut "Meatballs" (see p. 187), or bite-size pieces of fish or chicken (making sure these are cooked through) on the second step.

COMFORTING CREAMY TOMATO SOUP

This perfect creamy tomato soup is potent with antioxidants. Tomatoes are a great source of vitamin C, potassium, folate, and vitamin K, which all help to boost the immune system and reduce anxiety. They also contain lycopene, a plant nutrient said to help alleviate anxiety.[1] Furthermore, the lycopene in cooked tomatoes is more bioavailable than in raw tomatoes.[2] Enjoy the soup with a healthy sandwich for dipping.

Total time: 30 minutes • Makes 3 servings

Ingredients:

One 28-ounce can whole tomatoes in juice

5 large tomatoes

15 cherry tomatoes

8 cups filtered water

1 celery rib, roughly chopped

¼ small onion, roughly chopped

1 garlic clove

1 teaspoon dried parsley

1 teaspoon dried thyme

1 tablespoon honey

Juice from 1 lemon

¼ teaspoon salt

¼ teaspoon black pepper

2 tablespoons MCT oil

2 tablespoons extra-virgin olive oil

¼ cup organic cream or coconut cream, optional

1 bay leaf

¼ cup organic cheese shreds or vegan shreds, optional

Fresh herbs, for serving

Avocado slices, for serving

Actions:

1. Place all the ingredients except the bay leaf, cheese, fresh herbs, and avocados in a blender. Puree until smooth. Taste. Season with more salt and pepper, if desired.

2. Add the raw soup blend to a pot with the bay leaf, and bring to a boil. Boil over medium-high heat for 10 minutes, then reduce the heat to low and simmer for another 10 minutes.

3. Serve the soup topped with fresh herbs, cheese, and avocado slices.

Tips:

*   You can enjoy this soup raw if you like—or cook it! That's the beauty of this recipe. (If served raw, omit the bay leaf.)

*   This soup also can be substituted as a sauce whenever you're cooking ground beef, spaghetti, lasagna, or any other recipe that calls for pasta sauce.

GROUNDING LENTIL SOUP WITH AVOCADO AND GINGER

Lentils, whether brown, green, yellow, red, or black, are rich in iron and folate and excellent sources of protein. They are packed with health-promoting polyphenols, a group of plant metabolites with potent antioxidant properties that protect us against various chronic diseases induced by oxidative stress, like anxiety. Evidence on dietary polyphenols has emerged that shows they play a prominent role in the prevention of degenerative diseases. Lentils are antioxidant, anti-obesity, cholesterol-reducing, anti-inflammatory, and anticancer.[3] Lentils are also quite low in calories while still making us feel nice and satisfied, because one cup has 15 grams of dietary fiber (both soluble and insoluble). Oh yeah—and they taste delicious!

Total time: 50 minutes • Makes 4 servings

Ingredients:

5 tablespoons extra-virgin olive oil

1 yellow onion, chopped

3 garlic cloves, chopped

½-inch piece of ginger, grated

2 teaspoons cumin powder

1 teaspoon dried thyme

1 teaspoon dried sage

1 teaspoon dried oregano

1 teaspoon turmeric powder

⅛ teaspoon cayenne pepper

1 teaspoon sea salt

¼ teaspoon black pepper

6 cups filtered water

1½ cups uncooked lentils, any color

3 celery stalks, cut into ¼-inch slices

1 carrot, cut into ¼-inch circles

Juice of 1 lemon

¼ cup chopped fresh cilantro

Toppings:

Extra-virgin olive oil, for drizzling

Salt and cayenne pepper, to taste

Fresh cilantro

Sliced avocado

Actions:

1. Heat the oil in a large pot. Add the onion and garlic and sauté over medium heat until golden brown, about 4 minutes.

2. Add the ginger and stir-fry for 1 minute. Add the cumin, thyme, sage, oregano, and turmeric powder and stir-fry for an additional minute. Add the cayenne, salt, and black pepper and stir-fry an additional minute, until the spices are fragrant.

3. Stir in the water, lentils, celery, and carrot and bring to a boil over high heat. Reduce the heat to medium-low, cover, and simmer the soup for 30 minutes, or until the lentils are soft.

4. Stir in the lemon juice and cilantro. Serve drizzled with extra-virgin olive oil and sprinkled with additional salt or cayenne pepper to taste. Top with fresh cilantro and avocado slices.

Tips:

- Serve with wild rice or quinoa.

- For a smoother, less chunky soup, puree the mixture in a blender after cooking.

- Some lentils are smaller than others and will require less cooking time.

Variations:

Tomato-Lentil Soup: Add 2 chopped tomatoes and 1 tablespoon tomato paste when adding the water.

Curry-Lentil Soup: Add 1½ tablespoons curry powder.

BASIC MASON JAR SALAD FORMULA

The formula for a mason jar salad is very simple. Basically, you are going to grab your mason jar and fill it up with your salad of choice, but in a specific order. Have fun creating vibrant layers when you make one of these.

- Start with your salad dressing on the bottom to keep the rest of the salad ingredients from getting soggy.

- Add the "wet ingredients," things like cucumbers, red peppers, and tomatoes. You can also incorporate fruits like strawberries and blackberries in this layer.

- Add your solid, heavier vegetables like carrots, chickpeas, broccoli, snap peas, beans, or cauliflower.

- Add your dry ingredients, including any nuts and seeds.

- Add your protein, such as bean or lentil pasta, meat, chicken, or egg.

- On the very top, add your lightest ingredients: dark leafy greens (e.g., lettuce, kale, spinach), fresh herbs, and sprouts. This will ensure the leaves don't get squished.

- When you are ready to eat, shake up the jar, and that's it—you'll have a salad in a jar! You can either tip it into a bowl or eat it straight from the jar.

When you are enjoying a salad, visualize that you are eating the rainbow. This has become a popular concept even among some medical doctors. Not only does it boost our mood because of the color therapy, but it has some deeper science to it. Christiane Northrup, M.D., advises: "Think color and you'll be on the right path, because the deep pigments in these foods contain powerful antioxidants. Go for broccoli; leafy green vegetables; berries; red, yellow, and green peppers; and tomatoes, and vary your choices through the seasons."[4]

Make Your Own Homemade Salad Dressing ... Forever!

I don't see any reason at all for us to buy regular salad dressings from the store. Frankly, it's a waste of money and we can make our own that taste even better using ingredients that are actually good for us. Conventional salad dressings have so many unnecessary ingredients, like genetically modified soybean oil, sugar, modified food starch, MSG, disodium guanylate, disodium inosinate, EDTA, and more. *Eww*, what a toxic mess and monstrous concoction for an anxious nervous system to have to deal with! Nobody ever says, "Let's go out to the garden and get some disodium guanylate and EDTA to put in our salad dressing." These salad dressings should come with a warning label that reads: "neurotoxic."

It's much better to make your own, and you can keep it in a jar in the fridge, where it will last for months!

BASIC SALAD DRESSING OR VINAIGRETTE

The basic premise of a salad dressing is combining an oil and an acid, which can be either lemon juice or vinegar. If you have those two ingredients on hand, you can always make your own dressing for tastier and more exciting salads. Then, of course, you can add other ingredients for all kinds of different flavors.

Total time: 5 minutes • Makes ⅓ cup dressing

Ingredients:

⅓ cup oil: extra-virgin olive, coconut, MCT, or avocado

2 tablespoons apple cider vinegar or balsamic vinegar (just make sure the balsamic doesn't contain white sugar or sulfites)

1 tablespoon fresh lemon juice

Sea salt and pepper, optional

Actions:

Add all the ingredients to a bowl and whisk until well combined. Season with sea salt and pepper, if desired.

Tip:

- Refrigerated in an airtight container or jar, this base salad dressing lasts for up to two months.

- Coconut oil is solid at temperatures below 76°F. Care must be taken when incorporating the oil at lower temperatures, and it's best eaten immediately rather than stored in the fridge.

Variations:

Asian Dressing: Add 3 tablespoons amino acids, 1 tablespoon sesame oil, 2 tablespoons honey, 1 tablespoon chopped fresh cilantro, 1 tablespoon toasted sesame seeds, and 2 diced scallions.

Caesar Salad Dressing: Add ¼ teaspoon mustard powder, 2 tablespoons nutritional yeast, ½ teaspoon honey, 1 teaspoon minced garlic, ¼ teaspoon salt, and ¼ teaspoon pepper.

Cheesy Dressing: Add 1 tablespoon nutritional yeast and ½ teaspoon sea salt.

Citrus Salad Dressing: Add the juice of 1 orange and 1 grapefruit.

Creamy Avocado Dressing: Add 1 seeded and peeled avocado, and either mash it or mix the dressing in a blender.

Garlic Salad Dressing: Add 2 teaspoons minced garlic or 1 teaspoon garlic powder.

Ginger Salad Dressing: Add 1-inch piece of ginger, minced.

Honey Mustard Dressing: Add 2 tablespoons honey, 1 tablespoon mustard powder, 1 teaspoon minced garlic, ¼ teaspoon sea salt, and ¼ teaspoon black pepper.

Hummus Salad Dressing: Add 2 tablespoons hummus.

Lime Vinaigrette: Use lime instead of lemon and add a bit of honey, if you want to make your dressing sweet.

Mango Salad Dressing: Add 1 peeled and seeded mango, and either mash it or mix the dressing in a blender.

Mustard Vinaigrette: Add 1 teaspoon minced garlic, 1 tablespoon mustard, ¼ teaspoon black pepper, and ¼ teaspoon salt.

Roasted Sunflower Seed Dressing: Add 2 tablespoons organic SunButter and mix until the dressing is smooth and creamy.

Sesame Ginger Dressing: Add 1 tablespoon toasted sesame seeds, 1 tablespoon grated ginger, 1 tablespoon organic SunButter, and 1 tablespoon tahini, and mix until the dressing is smooth.

Spicy Salad Dressing: Add ⅛ teaspoon cayenne pepper.

Sweet Salad Dressing: Add 1 tablespoon honey.

Tahini Salad Dressing: Add 2 tablespoons tahini.

Thai Curry Dressing: Add 2 tablespoons green or red curry paste.

Turmeric Salad Dressing: Add 1 teaspoon turmeric powder for extra health benefits.

GREEN SPROUT SALAD

This ultimate green salad is made from dark leafy greens, among the most powerful foods for reducing stress and anxiety. Built on a foundation of herbs, this salad is so simple yet really flavorful and refreshing. It is also ridiculously high in antioxidants and magnesium, so you will feel better immediately, I promise! Try this salad. What a powerful thing, to fill up on greens!

Total time: 15 minutes • Makes 1 serving

Ingredients:

1 avocado, cubed

1 cup fresh parsley leaves

1 small cucumber, sliced

1 cup fresh cilantro leaves

1 cup broccoli sprouts

¼ cup grated broccoli

1 lemon

1 tablespoon extra-virgin olive oil

Sea salt and pepper, to taste

Actions:

1. Add all the ingredients except the lemon, olive oil, and seasonings to a bowl. Toss until well combined.

2. Slice the lemon in half and squeeze lemon juice over the salad, then drizzle with olive oil. Season with salt and pepper, to taste.

GUACAMOLE GREENS CHICKEN SALAD

This is my favorite salad of late, and I like to call this the party salad. It makes me feel like I'm on the beach or at a party somewhere with people I love and enjoy. This is also my go-to salad when I do long days at the Complete Wellness center, the medical facility where I work in New York City, seeing patients one-on-one. This salad makes me excited about eating lunch and helps me stay energized until dinnertime. It has some Mexican flavors, featuring a lime vinaigrette and corn chips, and contains satisfying protein that comes from delightfully juicy baked chicken breast.

Here is a tip for grilling chicken breasts, a cooking hack that changed everything for me in regard to getting the juiciest chicken ever. Bake the chicken breast for a shorter time at a higher temperature. Baking a chicken breast for 15 to 20 minutes at 450°F will surely give you the juiciest breast you have ever eaten. Baking chicken for 30 minutes at 350°F or lower will make for dry meat unless you baste it every so often or slather it with oil.

Total time: 25 minutes • Makes 1 serving

Ingredients:

1 organic chicken breast
½ small head of lettuce, diced
¼ cup cherry tomatoes, halved
½ cucumber, sliced into rounds and then halved
½ carrot, grated
1 tablespoon diced red onion

1 tablespoon chopped fresh cilantro
½ avocado, mashed
2 tablespoons extra-virgin olive oil
Juice from 1 lime
Sea salt and pepper, to taste
½ cup organic corn chips or cassava chips

Actions:

1. Preheat the oven to 450°F. Place the chicken breast on an oiled baking tray and bake for 15 to 20 minutes until cooked through.

2. While the chicken roasts, make the salad by combining the lettuce, tomatoes, cucumber, carrot, onion, and cilantro in a bowl. Add the mashed avocado and toss well.

3. Whisk together the olive oil, lime juice, salt, and pepper and pour the mixture over the salad.

4. Slice the chicken or cut into bite-size cubes, and add to the salad. Also add the corn or cassava chips, toss well, and enjoy!

SUPERFOOD KALE SALAD

This is the recipe that converted me to loving salads. The creaminess of the avocado makes the kale softer and more enjoyable to eat, and the nutritional yeast gives it a cheese flavor. This ultimate comfort salad is abundant in protein and amino acids while being totally vegan.

Total time: 10 minutes • Makes 3 servings

Ingredients:

1 bunch kale, center ribs and stems removed (save the stems and ribs for juicing or eating later)

1 avocado

1 tablespoon apple cider vinegar

1½ tablespoons flaxseed oil

¾ teaspoon sea salt or 2 teaspoons amino acids

¼ cup nutritional yeast

2 tablespoons raw sunflower seeds

2 tablespoons raw or roasted pumpkin seeds

Actions:

1. Tear the kale leaves into small pieces and place in a large bowl.

2. Massage the avocado into the pieces of kale with your fingers, covering the kale thoroughly with avocado.

3. Add the remaining ingredients to the bowl and stir, or continue to massage the mixture with your fingers, until everything is well combined.

Tip:

For immune-boosting benefits, add 2 teaspoons garlic powder.

ORANGE ARUGULA AVOCADO SESAME SEED SALAD

This salad is the ideal delicious and refreshing antianxiety lunch. It's got the elements of the vibrant citrus, good healthy fats from the avocado, and the health benefits of the sesame seeds, which are high in iron. If your iron levels are ever low, sprinkle sesame seeds on your salads, soups, and eggs.

Total time: 10 minutes • Makes 2 servings

Ingredients:

For the salad:

1 orange, peeled and sliced

2 cups arugula, torn into pieces

1 thin slice of red onion

1 avocado, peeled and sliced

¾ cup snap peas

For the dressing:

1 teaspoon sesame seed oil

2 teaspoons extra-virgin olive oil

Dash of sea salt and pepper

Juice of ½ lemon

1 tablespoon orange juice

For the garnish:

2 tablespoons roasted sesame seeds

Fresh parsley

Fresh cilantro

½ cup broccoli spouts

Actions:

1. Assemble the salads on 2 plates in layers, starting with the orange slices, then adding the arugula, followed by the onion, avocado, and snap peas.

2. Make the dressing by whisking the ingredients together in a bowl and pour over each salad.

3. Finish by sprinkling the salads with the seeds, fresh herbs, and broccoli sprouts.

Tip:

If you want to add a protein, baked salmon is great with these flavors.

CHICKPEA CABBAGE SALAD

A lot of chopping goes into this recipe, so use it as a meditation exercise and enjoy it as kitchen therapy. This salad makes a delicious plant-based meal, with its comforting combination of chickpeas, brussels sprouts, cabbage, and sesame seed oil dressing. But if you like, you can top it with some Baked Walnut-Crusted Salmon (see p. 234), or break the salmon into pieces and toss together with the salad.

The powerful combination of chickpeas and cabbage makes this a brain power salad. Cabbage is packed with an impressive array of nutrients! It belongs to the cruciferous family of vegetables and, like its cousins broccoli and cauliflower, brims with antioxidants, fiber, and vitamin C. One cup of raw red cabbage contains 85 percent of our daily vitamin C requirement!

If one of your anxiety symptoms is insomnia, it may interest you to know that red cabbage was reported to have hypnotic effects in one scientific study, so it may help to induce a good sleep. Flavonoids found in red cabbage are the main chemical component responsible for this effect.[5]

Wow, talk about a super salad!

Total time: 30 minutes • Makes 4 servings

Ingredients:

For the salad:

½ small red cabbage, diced

8 brussels sprouts, grated

7 radishes, sliced and then cut in halves

1 cucumber, sliced and then cut in halves

½ cup diced fresh parsley

¼ red onion, diced

⅓ cup minced dill

½ cup broccoli sprouts

2 cups or 1 14-oz. can chickpeas, drained

For the dressing:

3 tablespoons sesame seed oil

3 tablespoons extra-virgin olive oil

Juice of 1 lemon

1 tablespoon apple cider vinegar

¼ teaspoon sea salt

¼ teaspoon black pepper

Actions:

1. Combine all the salad ingredients in a large bowl.
2. Make the dressing by whisking the ingredients together in a bowl, and pour over the salad. Divide the salad onto 4 plates.

Tip:

You can use sprouted chickpeas to keep more raw elements in the salad.

SPINACH SALAD WITH GRILLED CHICKEN, AVOCADO, AND WALNUTS

This salad is packed with ingredients to increase your neurotransmitters and fire up the brain with positive energy, while also satiating the body with protein and healthy fats. Spinach contains chlorophyll, which puts oxygen into the body and makes us feel more energized instantly. Apple cider vinegar gives the dressing a delicious tang and is also excellent for cleansing the body and improving digestive health. Thyme and rosemary are "genius" herbs that increase focus and stamina.

Total time: 25 minutes • Makes 4 servings

Ingredients:

For the salad:

1 pound organic chicken breasts
2 tablespoons olive or avocado oil
1 teaspoon dried thyme
1 teaspoon dried rosemary
6 cups spinach
1 avocado, sliced
¼ small red onion, sliced
⅓ cup walnuts, chopped
Red chili flakes or fresh red chili,
   diced (for garnish, optional)

For the dressing:

⅓ cup olive or avocado oil
2 tablespoons apple cider vinegar
1 tablespoon fresh lemon juice
¼ teaspoon sea salt
¼ teaspoon black pepper

Actions:

1. Coat chicken with oil, then sprinkle with thyme and rosemary. Let the chicken rest for 30 minutes at room temperate before grilling.

2. Preheat the gas grill to medium-high until the temperature reaches 400°F. Lightly grease grates with oil to prevent sticking. Add chicken, close lid, and cook for 8 minutes. Turn the chicken over and cook for 7 minutes more or until done. Let the chicken sit for 5 minutes before slicing.

3. Divide spinach, avocado, onion, and walnuts evenly between four plates. Then arrange the sliced chicken on the plates.

4. Whisk all the vinaigrette ingredients in a small bowl, then drizzle it over the salads. Garnish salads with chili, if desired.

Tip:

Instead of grilling, you can bake the chicken breast at 450°F for 15 to 20 minutes, or until the internal temperature reaches 160°F.

WALNUT-CRUSTED CHICKEN SALAD

This delicious salad tastes like you ordered it from your favorite café, and it's full of antianxiety ingredients.

Total time: 40 minutes • Makes 4 servings

Ingredients:

For the salad:

1 head of lettuce, sliced

½ cup grated broccoli

8 brussels sprouts, grated

1 cup broccoli sprouts

1 batch of Walnut-Crusted Chicken (see p. 236)

For the dressing:

Pick any salad dressing you like: The Basic Salad Dressing (see p. 208) is always a good choice, but the Honey Mustard Dressing and the Caesar Salad Dressing (see p. 209) are also excellent with this salad.

Actions:

1. Add the lettuce to a bowl. Grate in the broccoli and brussels sprouts, so you get a shaved greens effect.

2. Add the broccoli sprouts and then the salad dressing. Toss until well combined.

3. Cut the Walnut-Crusted Chicken into slices or bite-size cubes, and add to the salad. Enjoy!

Variation:

Walnut-Crusted Salmon: You can also make this salad with salmon if you prefer! Swap in a ½ or ¾ batch of Baked Walnut-Crusted Salmon (see p. 234) for the chicken.

CHAPTER 11

Fun Sides, Savory Snacks, Sensational Sauces, and Life-Changing Condiments

Quick and easy sides and snacks can be incredibly useful, especially if you have anxiety that is making you indecisive about what to eat. If you always have some healthy, nourishing, delicious snacks on standby, it may just uplift your mood right away knowing they are there.

A snack or a side dish can also become a meal! Enjoy the following recipes.

GARLIC MASHED POTATOES

This side is a scrumptious blend of potatoes with cauliflower. The potatoes are a concentrated source of vitamin C and potassium (more than any other vegetable per standard serving), so it is no wonder that potatoes are something we crave—they help boost our immune system! This dish adds cruciferous power as well.

Total time: 20 minutes • Makes 4 servings

Ingredients:

2 teaspoons sea salt, divided

4 medium organic white potatoes

½ large head of cauliflower

3½ tablespoons butter-flavored Nutiva Coconut Oil

½ teaspoon black pepper

2 tablespoons nutritional yeast

3 tablespoons milk

1 teaspoon minced garlic

For the garnish:

Fresh parsley or diced scallions

Actions:

1. Bring a large pot of water to a boil, making sure there is enough water to cover the potatoes by an inch. Add 1 teaspoon salt to the pot.

2. While the water is heating, peel the potatoes and chop them into ½-inch pieces. Add the potato chunks to the boiling water and continue to boil for 15 minutes.

3. Meanwhile, cut the cauliflower into ½-inch chunks. After the potatoes have been boiling for 15 minutes, add the cauliflower to the pot and cook for another 10 to 15 minutes, until both the potatoes and cauliflower are soft. Drain.

4. Add the remaining ingredients, including the reserved salt, to the pot and mash everything together until smooth and creamy—unless you like some chunks in your mash!

5. Top with fresh parsley or diced scallions and serve.

Tips:

- You can use butter from grass-fed cows instead of coconut oil.

- Use a plant-based milk instead of dairy milk to make this recipe vegan.

- Stir in cooked organic peas and corn after the potatoes are mashed.

ROASTED BRUSSELS SPROUTS AND BROCCOLI

Total time: 35 minutes • Makes 4 servings

Ingredients:

⅓ cup organic SunButter

¼ cup nutritional yeast

¼ cup extra-virgin olive oil or avocado oil

1 teaspoon sea salt

½ teaspoon dried thyme

1 head of broccoli, cut into bite-size pieces

2 cups brussels sprouts, halved

¼ cup walnut pieces

Actions:

1. Preheat the oven to 325°F.

2. Mix together the SunButter, nutritional yeast, oil, salt, and thyme in a large bowl. Whisk or combine well. Stir in the broccoli, brussels sprouts, and walnuts until fully coated.

3. Arrange the mixture on baking tray. Bake for 20 to 25 minutes, until golden brown.

THAI SAUTÉED GREENS WITH GARLIC AND SWEET CHILI LIME

This recipe was inspired by a sunny Australian beach day and has a farm-to-table vibe. It makes a great side dish with chicken or fish, or you can halve the recipe and eat it all as a main dish.

Total time: 25 minutes • Makes 4 servings as a side dish (2 servings as a main)

Ingredients:

3 tablespoons extra-virgin olive oil

2 teaspoons sesame seed oil

4 garlic cloves, thinly sliced

1 cup broccoli rabe

½ cup bok choy

1 cup snow peas

1 cup spinach

1 tablespoon amino acids

1 tablespoon apple cider vinegar

3 tablespoons honey or maple syrup

1 red hot chili pepper, thinly sliced, or 1 teaspoon red chili flakes

Coarse sea salt, to taste

1 lime, cut into 4 wedges

Actions:

1. Heat both oils in a skillet over medium heat. Add the garlic and keep stirring for 2 minutes.

2. Add the broccoli rabe, bok choy, and snow peas and toss them with the oil. Once the vegetables have wilted a bit, add the spinach.

3. Add the amino acids, apple cider vinegar, and honey and toss to combine.

4. Add the chili pepper and sea salt. The greens are done when the broccoli rabe stems are tender.

5. Serve with lime wedges.

GONE CRACKERS

Got anxiety? Let's own it! Jokes aside, this is a fun cracker recipe that tastes delicious and, as you can see by looking at the ingredients, is clearly healthy.

Total time: 20 minutes to assemble, 12 hours to set in refrigerator, and 15 to 20 hours to dehydrate • Makes 20 crackers (6 servings)

Ingredients:

3 cups ground flaxseeds

1 cup roasted or raw sunflower seeds

2 tablespoons minced onion or 3 tablespoons onion powder

2 tablespoons toasted or raw sesame seeds

1 tablespoon minced garlic or 2 tablespoons garlic powder

2 teaspoons cumin powder

1 teaspoon chili powder

1 teaspoon sea salt

1 teaspoon cayenne pepper

½ teaspoon turmeric

½ cup filtered water

Actions:

1. Add all the dry ingredients to a food processor or high-speed blender and blend until a fine, flour-like consistency is achieved.

2. Add the water a little at a time and mix until a batter forms. Cover and allow the batter to set in the fridge for 12 hours.

3. *Dehydrator method:* Spread a ⅛-inch layer of batter on nonstick dehydrator sheets and dehydrate at 100°F for 15 to 20 hours.

4. *Oven method:* Spread a layer of batter on nonstick baking paper or a baking sheet lightly greased with coconut oil and place in the oven at 180°F for 2 to 4 hours, or until crisp and dry, checking frequently for doneness.

5. Cut or break the cracker sheet into pieces, and then store in an airtight container in the fridge for up to 8 weeks.

Tips:

- Serve these crackers with hummus, tahini, pesto sauce, and/or Cashew Cheese (see p. 223).

- This dough can be used as the base for a raw pizza or tacos! Simply mold the dough into the desired shape and size for your pizza crust or taco shells before dehydrating.

HUMMUS

The good news is that chickpeas reduce stress and anxiety, so you can go ahead and enjoy hummus as a snack with fresh organic vegetables, like carrot, celery, and cucumber sticks, any time you want. Hummus may be substituted for mayonnaise in sandwiches and for sour cream or butter on a baked potato. In a 2007 assessment of peer-reviewed studies on how to increase serotonin in the human brain without drugs, chickpeas were among the few foods recommended because of their high tryptophan content.[1]

An article in the journal *Nutrients* describes how consumers of chickpeas and/or hummus have been shown to have higher nutrient intakes of dietary fiber, polyunsaturated (aka good) fatty acids, vitamins A, E, and C, folate, magnesium, potassium, and iron as compared to nonconsumers. Hummus eaters have also been shown to have higher Healthy Eating Index 2005 scores, which may be due to "hummus' higher Naturally Nutrient Rich (NNR) score as compared to other dips and spreads."[2]

With chickpeas as the primary ingredient in hummus, which is then paired with fresh organic vegetables, you get a powerful antianxiety snack, plus a nutritious way to obtain the recommended daily serving of legumes. In this recipe, I have omitted the classic ingredient tahini (sesame paste) in favor of a small amount of extra-virgin olive oil paired with sesame seeds to reduce the fat content.

Total time: 10 minutes • Makes 4 to 6 servings

Ingredients:

One 14-ounce can chickpeas	1 tablespoon lemon juice
¼ cup chickpea water from the can	2 tablespoons sesame seeds
1 tablespoon extra-virgin olive oil	1 teaspoon sea salt
3 garlic cloves	Dash of turmeric powder

Actions:

Put all the ingredients in your food processor and blend until smooth.

Tip:

Get creative and add sunflower seeds, organic SunButter, or hempseeds.

CASHEW CHEESE

This plant-based alternative to cheese makes a great spread for pasta or a dip for veggies! Cashews contain anacardic acids and have been proven to have an anxiolytic effect.[3]

Total time: 10 minutes • Makes 8 servings

Ingredients:

2 cups cashews

2 tablespoons nutritional yeast

Juice of 1 small lemon (3 to 5 tablespoons)

½ teaspoon sea salt

½ cup filtered water

Actions:

Put all the ingredients in a food processor. Blend until the mixture is smooth, adding more water if a softer cheese is desired.

Tips:

- For a smoother, creamier cheese, soak the cashews for 4 hours.
- For a nut-free version, use hempseeds, pumpkin seeds, or sunflower seeds instead of cashews.
- This recipe also works well with almonds, macadamia nuts, walnuts, or Brazil nuts.
- For a cheesier flavor, add more nutritional yeast, to taste. You can also make this recipe without nutritional yeast.
- For spice, add a dash of cayenne pepper or chili flakes.

Variations:

Raw "Parmesan" Cheese: Add 3 additional tablespoons nutritional yeast to the mixture and spread to ¼-inch thick on a dehydrator tray. Place in a food dehydrator for 12 hours. It will crumble easily when you're ready to use it.

Garlic Cashew Cheese: Add 1 or more garlic cloves before blending.

Pesto Cashew Cheese: Add 1 cup fresh basil leaves before blending.

Thyme Cashew Cheese: Add 1 teaspoon of fresh thyme before blending.

BLUEBERRY CHIA SEED JAM

This jam will last up to two months in the refrigerator and six months in the freezer.

Total time: 20 minutes • Makes 12 servings (about 2 tablespoons per serving)

Ingredients:

2 cups blueberries

1 cup filtered water

¼ cup chia seeds

¼ cup maple syrup or honey

Actions:

1. Place all the ingredients in a pot and bring to a boil.

2. Reduce the heat to a simmer and stir constantly so the chia seeds do not burn on the bottom of the pot.

3. When the mixture has thickened and the fruit is entirely broken down (about 10 minutes), allow to cool and then place in a glass jar to cool completely before placing the jam in the fridge. Once it has cooled, the jam is ready to eat, but it will set more if you refrigerate it overnight.

Variations:

Strawberry Chia Seed Jam: Use strawberries.

Blackberry Chia Seed Jam: Use blackberries.

Raspberry Chia Seed Jam: Use raspberries.

Mixed Berry Chia Seed Jam: Use ½ cup each of strawberries, blackberries, raspberries, and blueberries.

WALNUT BUTTER

Walnuts have the highest amount of antioxidants of any nut or seed on earth! The idea here is to roast some walnuts and then blend them into a smooth nut butter that is delicious on its own as a snack or with fruit like strawberries. It can also be added as a brain-health booster to a smoothie, a salad, or desserts like the Genius Chocolate Balls (see p. 246). Because walnuts are relatively high in fat as compared to other nuts, walnut butter comes out much smoother than almond or cashew butter.

Total time: 15 minutes • Makes 24 servings (about 2 tablespoons per serving)

Ingredients:

3 cups raw, unsalted walnuts

Sea salt, to taste (optional)

Actions:

1. Preheat the oven to 300°F. Place the walnuts on baking paper on a baking tray, then place in the oven for 12 minutes, or until just golden brown. Watch them carefully to make sure they don't burn.

2. Place the baked walnuts in a food processor with the salt, if using, and mix until completely smooth. You may need to stop and scrape down the sides of your processor bowl and reblend to get the consistency just right. Store your Walnut Butter in a jar in the refrigerator.

Tips:

- A food processor works better than a blender for making nut butters.
- For different flavors, add spices like cardamom, cinnamon, and nutmeg, to taste.
- For sweetness, add honey or coconut sugar.

Variations:

Chocolate Walnut Butter: Add 2 tablespoons cacao powder.

Walnut-Pecan Butter: Use 1½ cups walnuts and 1½ cups pecans.

CHAPTER 12

Meals for Fish and Meat Eaters

This section is for the fish and meat eaters among us. All of these recipes are dairy- and gluten-free and incorporate high-quality, nutrient-rich ingredients to nourish you fully. These are hearty, delicious options that will balance the flora in your gut, take care of your brain, and calm your nervous system. Don't be surprised if you start to feel much better after eating these dishes and making them part of your new way of eating. These recipes have strong potential to reduce stress and anxiety while lifting your mood and making you feel fulfilled and excited.

First, a few things about the quality of the meat we choose to consume. One way we can protect ourselves from symptoms of anxiety is to eat organic meat from ethically raised animals. Unfortunately, factory farming is widespread and puts low-quality meat from ill-treated animals on our grocery store shelves. A meta-analysis of multiple studies reported in *British Journal of Nutrition* showed that there are significant and nutritionally meaningful composition differences between organic and nonorganic meats.[1]

The best types of meat for your body to metabolize incorporate the following properties:

- Organic (this means the animal or bird eats organic produce as its feed)

- Grass-fed (which comes from cattle that are free-grazing)
- Non-GMO
- Local, from a farm you trust
- Wild-caught (fish)
- Poultry that is free-range or pasture-raised

It is incredibly important to opt for organic grass-fed beef. Personally, I refuse to eat beef unless it is grass-fed and organic. Factory farming that produces conventional meat is not only polluting the environment, it is also distributing meat that is full of contaminants we don't want in our bodies, as well as a preservative that is sometimes added to keep the meat looking "pink" for as long as possible on the store shelf after butchering. Grass-fed beef that is also organic is from cows that were treated better and given a higher-quality feed, which also makes it higher in key nutrients, including antioxidant vitamins and conjugated linoleic acid (CLA), a beneficial fat that has been said to improve immunity and has anti-inflammatory properties.[2]

It's the same with chicken and eggs. Organic chicken is said to contain 38 percent more heart-healthy omega-3 fatty acids than factory-farmed chicken.[3] Eating organic chicken may also lower your risk of getting food poisoning: In a 2010 study, fewer than 6 percent of organic birds were infected with salmonella, compared with almost 39 percent of conventional ones.[4]

People always ask, "Is it really worth it to buy organic?" Yes. And "Just because there is an organic label, does it really mean it is?" Yes, the organic label guarantees certain standards.

If you are really interested, I would suggest visiting a conventional chicken farm and then an organic one. This way, you will see things with your own eyes that will make you want to buy only organic forever.

Here are some of the standards organic chicken farmers must adhere to. They are prohibited from using:

- Sewage sludge as fertilizer

- Synthetic chemicals not approved by the National Organic Program of the U.S. Department of Agriculture (USDA)

- Genetically modified organisms (GMOs)—any plant, animal, or microorganism that has been altered through genetic engineering—in their poultry production process

Chicken labeled as "natural" does not necessarily meet those standards. ("Natural" is more of a marketing term rather than a regulated label.) Furthermore, each country has its own standards for what is considered "organic." Even so, it is always safer to purchase certified organic chicken.

The same goes with purchasing eggs. The healthiest kind are labeled "organic pasture-raised." Free-range eggs are better than caged eggs, yes; however, organic eggs are even cleaner and far superior nutritionally to free-range.

Consuming only wild-caught fish is also an important choice you can make that may impact your anxiety levels positively. As I mentioned earlier, there is great importance to avoiding farmed fish and seafood.

If you are concerned about getting too much mercury from fish, try drinking 1 teaspoon of bentonite clay mixed in 2 cups of water. Bentonite clay binds with heavy metals in the body, including mercury and other pollutants in our air and water, and helps us to eliminate them from the body. Furthermore, if you are consuming chlorophyll daily in dark leafy greens or liquid chlorophyll supplementation (see "Chlorophyll" section on p. 82), your cells are protected from heavy metal damage.[5] It would be unlikely to contract heavy metal poisoning from eating seafood.

With regard to purchasing seafood, it might be best to go to a local market and see what is local and wild-caught—unless, of course, your area is landlocked or surrounded by toxic oceans. If fish has been flown into your area, ask where it came from and how it was fished.

GRASS-FED BEEF BURRITOS/TACOS

What I love about this recipe is that you can choose to make it a burrito or a taco depending on whether you wrap it or shell it! Choose an organic soft tortilla for a burrito, and a non-GMO corn taco shell for a taco. Either way the result can be a delicious feast for just you alone or for an entire family. The spices are all super for the brain and delicious.

You can even do a lettuce wrap for a burrito if you want to reduce carbs. And you can choose a different meat, too! Chicken, fish, and shrimp also make great burrito and taco fillers.

For a vegan option, you can use beans instead of meat.

Total time: 25 minutes • Makes 4 servings

Ingredients:

2 tablespoons extra-virgin olive oil

1 teaspoon turmeric powder

¼ teaspoon black pepper

1 pound organic grass-fed ground beef

1 small yellow onion, chopped

2 large garlic cloves, diced

1½ teaspoons ground cumin

½ teaspoon paprika

¼ teaspoon sea salt

¼ teaspoon pepper

1 teaspoon chili powder or ¼ teaspoon cayenne pepper, optional

4 tortillas, 4 lettuce wraps, or 8 taco shells

Fillings (your choice):

¾ cup organic sour cream or vegan sour cream

1 cup nutritional yeast

½ cup grated carrot

1 cup chopped lettuce

1 avocado, cubed

1 pepper, diced

Fresh chopped cilantro

1 handful of broccoli sprouts

16 ounces black beans (soaked, cooked, soft)

Actions:

1. Heat the oil in a large frying pan over medium heat. Add turmeric and black pepper. Sauté for 1 minute or until sizzling. Add the beef and cook for 3 to 4 minutes or until it turns brown, stirring frequently.

2. Add the onion, garlic, cumin, paprika, salt, pepper, and chili powder, if using, to the meat and stir. Cook for 7 minutes, or until the vegetables are tender and the flavors are well combined.

3. Place ¼ cup of meat into each tortilla, or 2 tablespoons into a taco shell, and then add your fillings of choice.

GRASS-FED BEEF BURGERS

For an Australian like me, a burger with the "lot" means a burger with everything! Try your burger with the lot, or add just a few of these extras for a boost of amino acids, protein, antioxidants, omega-3 fats, or other nutrients. It's quite fun to build a huge, delicious, juicy burger with the lot.

Total time: 20 minutes • Makes 4 servings

Ingredients:

For the patties:

1 pound organic ground beef

2 eggs, beaten

1 cup almond meal

1 teaspoon dried sage

1 teaspoon sea salt

½ teaspoon turmeric powder

¼ teaspoon cumin

¼ teaspoon dried rosemary

½ teaspoon black pepper

¼ cup extra-virgin coconut oil or avocado oil (for frying)

Even more "lot," your choice:

Caramelized onions

Slices of tomato

Pickles

4 organic or gluten-free hamburger buns, optional

The "lot":

4 lettuce leaves

4 slices of organic cheese or vegan cheese

4 fried eggs

4 slices of beetroot

4 slices of pineapple

4 pieces of organic turkey bacon

4 slices of avocado

¼ cup broccoli sprouts

Your choice of sauces:

Organic ketchup (not sweetened with sugar or corn syrup, please)

Mayonnaise

Mustard

Actions:

1. Place all the ingredients for the patties except the coconut oil in a bowl. Mix until thoroughly combined, then form 4 patties by hand.

2. Heat the oil in a large frying pan over medium heat. When the pan is hot, place the patties in it.

3. Allow the patties to cook until the undersides have browned, then flip them over. Cook until desired doneness is achieved, about 4 to 8 minutes per side.

4. Serve on hamburger buns, if desired, topped with the "lot" and your choice of sauce.

Tip:

Serve with Cauliflower Cheese Fries (see p. 199) or Hash Browns (see p. 184).

SPAGHETTI AND GRASS-FED MEATBALLS

These meatballs are also tasty the next day as leftovers and can save you some prep time for tomorrow's lunch or dinner. This recipe includes a homemade tomato pasta sauce; however, you can always use an organic store-bought tomato sauce if you want to save some time.

Total time 25 minutes • Makes 4 servings

Ingredients:

For the sauce:

2 tablespoons extra-virgin olive oil or avocado oil

1 small yellow onion, diced

2 garlic cloves, chopped

5 large organic tomatoes, chopped into bite-size cubes

1 container of cherry tomatoes, halved

1 tablespoon tapioca flour

½ teaspoon sea salt

¼ teaspoon ground black pepper

½ teaspoon dried oregano

For the spaghetti:

1 box gluten-free Explore Cuisine Chickpea Spaghetti (or another brand)

For the meatballs:

2 tablespoons extra-virgin
  coconut oil

2 eggs

1 pound organic grass-fed
  ground beef

1 teaspoon sea salt

½ teaspoon pepper

½ teaspoon dried sage

½ teaspoon dried oregano

½ teaspoon dried parsley

¼ teaspoon turmeric powder

½ teaspoon dried rosemary

For the garnish:

1 handful of fresh parsley

1 handful of broccoli sprouts

Actions:

1. *Start with making the tomato sauce:* Heat the oil in a pot over medium heat. Add the onion and garlic and sauté a few minutes, until the onion turns translucent, stirring occasionally. Add the tomatoes, 1 cup water, tapioca, and spices. Bring the mixture to a boil, then reduce the heat to medium. Cook for 15 minutes more, stirring occasionally, until you have a beautiful tomato sauce. It'll be all melded together with some chunks and juicy looking. Remove from heat.

2. *Make the chickpea spaghetti:* Cook per the box instructions.

3. *Make the meatballs:* Heat the oil in a frying pan over medium heat. Meanwhile, beat the eggs in a bowl and add the ground beef to them. Use your hands to combine the ingredients well, then add the spices and mix again.

4. Roll the meat mixture into balls your desired size. Add the meatballs to the frying pan and cook until desired doneness, turning occasionally to brown on all sides.

5. *Assemble the bowls:* Place the pasta in 4 bowls, then divide the meatballs evenly and top with the tomato sauce. Garnish with fresh parsley and broccoli sprouts!

BAKED WALNUT-CRUSTED SALMON

Walnuts and salmon combine for an omega-3 powerhouse meal! I like using parchment paper for baking the fish, but you can thinly coat the baking sheet with oil instead.

Total time: 35 minutes • Makes 4 servings

Ingredients:

1 tablespoon coconut oil (optional, if not using parchment paper)

1 cup walnuts, processed to a chunky meal in a blender

1 teaspoon dried sage

½ teaspoon sea salt

2 tablespoons fresh dill, minced

1 teaspoon dried thyme

1½ pounds skinless salmon, cut into 4 pieces

1 handful of broccoli sprouts

Actions:

1. Preheat the oven to 375°F.

2. Line a baking sheet with parchment paper or a thin coating of coconut oil.

3. Mix the walnut meal, sage, sea salt, dill, and thyme in a bowl. Press each salmon fillet into the walnut mixture to coat top and bottom. Transfer the salmon to the prepared baking sheet.

4. Bake for 7 minutes. Check to see if the salmon is flaky and cooked to your liking; bake for up to another 7 minutes, depending on thickness.

5. Serve with a sprinkle of broccoli sprouts.

Tip:

Serve the salmon with Green Sprout Salad (see p. 210) and/or Garlic Mashed Potatoes (see p. 218).

Rosemary, the Superherb

Science has shown us that rosemary is both an anxiolytic and antidepressant![6] Rosemary is also said to help with memory and focus.[7] That qualifies rosemary as officially being a brain superherb! After doing research into the benefits of rosemary, I decided to grow a small pot of it on the windowsill in my apartment so I can add it fresh to foods and also enjoy its heavenly aroma. I encourage you to do the same. If you already grow rosemary at home, you have another therapeutic food in your surroundings ready to help relieve anxiety!

It has been said that just smelling rosemary gives the brain a boost and reduces stress; so whenever you see a fresh rosemary plant, take the opportunity to smell it. If you crush a few spikes between your hands, their scent will release.[8]

HONEY ROSEMARY CHICKEN

This quick and easy recipe is high in antioxidants from the honey and rosemary. It's a protein-laden way of satisfying a craving for something sweet.

Total time: 10 minutes • Makes 3 servings

Ingredients:

¼ cup extra-virgin coconut oil, for cooking

1 pound chicken breasts, cubed

1 teaspoon garlic powder

1 bunch fresh rosemary, destemmed; or ¼ cup dried rosemary

5 tablespoons raw honey

Actions:

1. Heat the oil in a frying pan over medium-high heat, then add the chicken.
2. Sprinkle the chicken with garlic powder and rosemary, then drizzle 1 tablespoon honey over it as it cooks.
3. Cook the chicken until done, roughly 7 minutes, turning so all sides are browned.
4. Serve the chicken with the remaining ¼ cup of honey drizzled on top.

Tips:
- This is a great recipe to use if you want to fire up the grill. It's fun to substitute rosemary stems for traditional wooden or metal skewers.
- Wrap the chicken in lettuce leaves to make some delicious wraps.

WALNUT-CRUSTED CHICKEN

This recipe is absolutely divine. The crunch of the nuts combined with the soft, succulent meat can win anyone over to the "healthier" side. Eat this when you are craving fried chicken. Unlike the toxic conventional version of fried chicken, this crust of turmeric and black pepper makes the dish anti-inflammatory—a major upgrade for when you want to enjoy chicken tenders!

Total time: 30 minutes • Makes 4 servings

Ingredients:

⅓ cup walnut meal

½ cup almond flour

1½ tablespoons turmeric powder

¼ teaspoon sea salt

¼ teaspoon black pepper

2 eggs

1 pound boneless, skinless chicken breasts

1 tablespoon extra-virgin coconut oil

1 handful of broccoli sprouts, for garnish

Actions:

1. Preheat the oven to 450°F.
2. Add the walnut meal, almond flour, turmeric, salt, and pepper to a bowl and mix until well combined.
3. Beat the eggs in a separate bowl.
4. Cut the chicken into tenders. Dip the tenders into the egg and then into the breading, turning until they're coated well on all sides.
5. Oil a baking tray and then place the chicken on it. Bake for 15 to 20 minutes.
6. Serve garnished with a sprinkle of broccoli sprouts and a side salad.

THAI CHICKEN PIZZA

Is it pizza night yet? Try this delicious pizza with a Thai-inspired sauce. However, instead of the usual peanut flavors, we're substituting roasted sunflower seed butter to give it more antianxiety power.

Total time: 1 hour • Makes 4 servings

Ingredients:

⅓ cup organic SunButter

3 tablespoons filtered water

1 tablespoon Bragg Liquid Aminos

1 tablespoon lime juice

1 tablespoon honey

1 garlic clove, crushed

1 teaspoon minced ginger

Red pepper flakes, to taste (optional)

1 tablespoon coconut oil, for frying

1 large organic chicken breast, diced

1 prepared pizza crust of your choice, either an organic crust or a gluten-free crust (perhaps cauliflower)

1 cup organic mozzarella cheese, shredded, or vegan "mozzarella" cheese, divided

3 scallions, chopped

½ cup roughly chopped cilantro

Actions:

1. Preheat the oven to 450°F.

2. Combine the SunButter, water, liquid aminos, lime juice, honey, garlic, ginger, and red pepper flakes (if using) in a saucepan. Cook over medium heat, stirring until the mixture is well combined.

3. Heat the oil in a frying pan over medium-high heat, then add the chicken. Halfway through cooking, pour in half the sauce, flip the chicken, and continue cooking until the chicken is done.

4. Place the pizza crust on a full sheet pan and spread the remaining sauce over the crust.

5. Top the crust with ¾ cup cheese, then add the chicken and scallions. Sprinkle the remaining ¼ cup cheese over the top of the pizza.

6. Bake the pizza for 12 to 15 minutes, or until the cheese is melted and the crust is fully cooked and crisp.

7. Top the pizza with fresh cilantro and red pepper flakes, if desired, and serve.

BAKED FISH WITH ROASTED VEGETABLES AND A SIDE OF YUCCA

I made baked fish and roasted vegetables so many times while I was writing this book. Some writing days seem very long, as you can imagine, especially when you get into a flow state. It's hard to stop when the creative juices are bubbling. On those days, I would go into the kitchen, grab some wild salmon and whatever veggies I had on hand, and throw this dish together for a rewarding dinner in less time than it takes to order delivery! This dish is high in protein, omega-3 fatty acids, and antioxidants to keep the brain powered.

Yucca pairs so heavenly with baked wild fish and roasted vegetables. You may also know this vegetable as cassava root or tapioca. Along with rice and corn, yucca is one of the primary sources of carbohydrates in the tropics. This superfood contains so much fiber, antioxidants, and saponin. It is known to reduce inflammation and lower blood pressure, thus reducing stress and anxiety.[9] Extracts from yucca are often sold in health food stores.

I first tried yucca after moving to New York. Served over rice and beans, it was so delicious and warming that it soon became my ultimate comfort food.

Total time: 35 minutes • Makes 1 serving

Ingredients:

For the yucca:

½ pound peeled yucca root, cut into 2-inch x ½-inch rectangles

1 tablespoon apple cider vinegar

½ teaspoon salt, plus more for seasoning, to taste

1 tablespoon butter-flavored Nutiva Coconut oil

For the fish and vegetables:

1 small carrot, chopped

¼ cup chopped broccoli

4 brussels sprouts, halved

½ yellow onion, cut into wedges

1 garlic clove, halved

1 piece of wild fish of your choice, such as salmon, tuna, or cod

3 tablespoons avocado oil

Sea salt and pepper, to taste

Actions:

1. Preheat the oven to 425°F.

2. Add the yucca, apple cider vinegar, and salt to a pot. (The vinegar imparts a subtle flavor and helps soften the yucca.) Add water until it comes to about an inch over the vegetables. Bring to a boil, then reduce the heat to medium and cook for another 25 to 30 minutes, until the yucca pieces are tender to your liking. (You should be able to pierce the yucca with a fork.) Drain the water and then toss the yucca with the coconut oil, if using, to give it a buttery flavor. Add salt to season.

3. While the yucca is cooking, chop up all the vegetables you will be roasting. Cut them into small, even pieces so they will cook more quickly.

4. Lightly oil the fish and place on a baking tray with the vegetables. Drizzle avocado oil over the vegetables, and season with salt and pepper, to taste. Place in the oven.

5. After 10 to 15 minutes, check the fish. If it's a smaller piece of fish, you may need to remove it from the oven and let it rest on a plate while the vegetables continue to cook. Vegetables may take 20 minutes depending on your oven, how well-cooked you like your fish and vegetables, and how small you've chopped the vegetables.

6. Serve the fish, veggies, and yucca on a plate together, and wow—enjoy! I wish I were there!

Tips:

- I always keep some fish in the freezer so I can easily make this quick meal! You don't even need to defrost the fish first; just add another 5 minutes or so to the cooking time.

- If you can't find yucca, you can substitute another root vegetable such as white potatoes—or simply make the fish and vegetables without another side dish.

TURKEY CHILI

Turkey is a high-quality protein that provides us with B vitamins, selenium, zinc, and phosphorus. Turkey is also known as the relaxation meat, or "sleepy meat," because it has a relaxing effect after we eat it, due to its high levels of tryptophan. Tryptophan is an essential amino acid and the sole precursor of peripherally and centrally produced serotonin.

Total time: 1 hour • Makes 6 servings

Ingredients:

1 tablespoon extra-virgin olive oil

1 large yellow onion, chopped

3 garlic cloves, chopped

1 medium red bell pepper, chopped

1 pound ground organic turkey

3 tablespoons chili powder

2 teaspoons cumin powder

1 teaspoon dried oregano

1 teaspoon paprika powder

¼ teaspoon cayenne pepper

½ teaspoon sea salt

¼ teaspoon ground black pepper

One 28-ounce can diced tomatoes or crushed tomatoes

1½ cups vegetable broth or filtered water

Two 15-ounce cans dark red kidney beans, rinsed and drained

2 carrots, chopped into small pieces

4 celery stalks, chopped into small pieces

One 15-ounce can organic sweet corn, rinsed and drained

Toppings (your choice):

Chili pepper, chopped

Organic cheese, shredded

Vegan cheese, shredded

Avocado slices

Tortilla chips

Fresh cilantro, chopped

Organic sour cream

Vegan sour cream

Fresh lime juice

Actions:

1. Add the oil to a large pot and set over medium heat. Add the onion, garlic, and red pepper and sauté for 5 to 7 minutes, stirring often.

2. Add in the ground turkey and cook until it is no longer pink, breaking it up into smaller pieces.

3. Add in the chili powder, cumin, oregano, paprika, cayenne, salt, and pepper; stir for 30 seconds until well combined.

4. Add in the tomatoes, broth, beans, carrots, celery, and corn. Bring to a boil, then reduce the heat and simmer for 35 to 45 minutes, or until the chili thickens.

5. Serve with the toppings of your choice and enjoy!

Tip:

For a slow-cooker turkey chili, repeat the same steps using a crockpot and cook on high for 3 hours or low for 6 hours.

DAIRY-FREE BUTTER CHICKEN CURRY

Delicious and buttery—but without the dairy—this recipe is also packed with anti-inflammatory elements in the spices. There's already turmeric in the curry powder, so you can adjust the amount of added turmeric to your liking. I recommend serving this curry on delicious gluten-free pasta rather than traditional rice to make this recipe lighter and grain-free.

Total time: 20 minutes • Makes 4 servings

Ingredients:

1 package Explore Cuisine chickpea fusilli

¼ cup Nutiva buttery coconut oil

1 small yellow onion, diced

1 teaspoon crushed garlic

1 teaspoon diced ginger

1 pound organic chicken breast, cubed

½ cup tomato paste

2.8 ounces of yellow curry paste (can also use red)

½ teaspoon turmeric

¼ teaspoon paprika

Chili powder, to taste (optional)

One 13.5-ounce can coconut cream

1 tablespoon SunButter

1 lime

⅓ cup fresh organic cilantro

Actions:

1. Cook the pasta according to package directions. Set aside.

2. Heat coconut oil in a frying pan over medium-high heat. Cook onion, garlic, and ginger for 5 minutes, until fragrant. Add chicken and stir-fry until white in color.

3. Stir in tomato sauce, curry paste, turmeric, paprika, chili (if using), coconut cream, and sunflower seed butter. Continue to simmer over low heat until chicken is cooked through, 4 to 5 minutes.

4. To serve, place chicken over pasta and garnish with squeeze of lime and fresh cilantro.

CHAPTER 13

Nutrient-Rich Desserts and Wholesome, Sweet Snacks

Desserts are a comfort food for many people. There's nothing wrong with eating desserts when you have anxiety. The problem is that most people are eating the wrong *type* of desserts. Indulging in desserts that are full of anxiety triggers, like refined sugars, refined gluten, additives, and nonorganic dairy, can wreak havoc on our bodies, especially our nervous systems. High-glycemic foods spike our blood sugar and can cause strong cravings for more just hours later.[1] This is why we impulsively grab that sweet treat, but before we know it we feel much worse than before. White table sugar and corn syrup trigger anxiety. Honey and fruits do not.

Researchers at Yale University demonstrated with MRI scans that the same reward circuits were activated in the brains of women shown pictures of milkshakes as are activated in addicts craving drugs or alcohol![2] By contrast, sweet treats with tastes, textures, and aromas that make us smile—especially chocolate— are top happiness triggers.

A key solution for lessening anxiety is to retrain your body to like desserts and snacks that are made from wholesome sweet ingredients instead of refined sugar. This is the only way to get your sweet fix without getting trapped in a vicious cycle of cravings followed by crashes.

The recipes here will help you break an addiction to sugary foods. These desserts incorporate items from the top 10 list of foods that reduce anxiety, like walnuts, cacao, avocados, strawberries, oranges, and sunflower seeds. We don't need to be afraid of desserts and sweet snacks if we eat the right kinds. You can satisfy your sweet tooth and nourish your brain at the same time.

It's remarkable that we can get nutrition from delicious-tasting desserts. My mind was blown when I first started to make these more than a decade ago. These are the desserts that helped me stop craving conventional sweets and refined sugars. They literally saved my health and changed my life.

These desserts all have tons of antioxidants, as they are mostly made with nuts and fruits, so they are anti-inflammatory and provide a lot of nutrients we need, including magnesium. They are all also free of gluten, dairy, and refined sugars. And, of course, they have no additives. When I do nutrition coaching, I always say, "Would you go out to your garden and grab preservative E60?" No, ha! Of course, you would not. There is no need for any additives in homemade desserts.

A bonus is that you may even achieve a healthy weight and body composition from eating these naturally sweet treats, like I did! See if you can never again eat white sugar or corn syrup, and instead opt for the kind of dessert staples you can have in your diet forever, as they will support long-lasting, sustainable health.

To reiterate, say no to conventional sweets but don't deprive yourself of good, wholesome sweets. You will be better off for it.

And never forget, you can always eat a piece of fruit to satisfy a craving for sweets. I believe we were meant to enjoy sweets, and that fruit is nature's candy, a gift from God. Depriving ourselves of desserts leads to us bingeing later. But if we eat healthy desserts, we can satisfy our bodies and get on with our day without experiencing any remorse.

If you have a nut allergy, opt for sunflower, pumpkin, and hempseeds. Chopped roasted sunflower seeds make a great alternative to chopped nuts. SunButter is an excellent alternative to peanut butter or almond butter. You can also use tigernuts to make a nut-free plant-based milk and/or gluten-free flour.

You may notice that there are a few brand-name items I include in my ingredient list. This is because there really aren't comparable products made by other companies at this time. For example, a few recipes call for Hu Chocolate Gems. As far as I know, Hu is the only company that makes chocolate bits containing coconut sugar instead of other sweeteners. You could make your own homemade sunflower seed butter, or you could use SunButter, which is the only mass-produced sunflower seed butter that is currently on the market that I am aware of. If you cannot find one of the brand-name products I recommend, then try the alternate ingredient I suggest. It's okay to be somewhat improvisational with these recipes as long as you are using wholesome ingredients.

Are you ready for something yummy? Read on!

GENIUS CHOCOLATE BALLS

This was the very first recipe I made when I started the Earth Diet. I love the original recipe; however, over the years I have added more superfoods, making it an even more powerful brain food!

Making healthy chocolate is easier than you may think. This recipe is probably simple enough for you to remember for the rest of your life without even looking. This chocolate can stay fresh in the fridge for two weeks and in the freezer for three months. The tapioca flour makes the chocolate balls very soft and delicious.

Total time: 10 minutes • Makes 12 balls

Ingredients:

1 cup nut meal (finely ground almonds or other nuts) or tigernut flour

¼ cup cacao powder

2 dates, seeded and diced

2 tablespoons honey

1 tablespoon MCT oil

1 tablespoon tapioca flour

¼ teaspoon vanilla

⅛ teaspoon salt

Actions:

1. Mix all the ingredients in a bowl, then roll the mixture into 1-inch balls with your hands. If the dough is sticky, add more nut meal. If the dough is too dry, add water.

2. These are ready to eat as soon as you roll them, but they can also be stored in the fridge or freezer for a different texture.

Tip:

For a cool-looking chocolate ball and some extra texture, roll them in hempseeds, goji berries, or chopped walnut pieces.

SMART COOKIES

These are my all-time favorite cookies! You can enjoy the cookie dough raw or baked. By dividing each batch, you can have the best of both worlds. I usually end up eating half of the dough raw. I roll half the dough into balls that I keep in the fridge, and bake the other half. These cookies are "clean" and vegan. Without eggs, they are safe to eat raw, yet completely moist and delicious. They are also packed with protein and micronutrients.

Whenever I am craving cookies, I know I can make these nourishing treats in a jiffy! Within 10 minutes, you, too, can be eating delicious cookies that melt in your mouth! I use butter-flavored Nutiva Coconut Oil in this recipe to give it the flavor of butter while still keeping it dairy-free.

Total time: 10 minutes • Makes 8 large cookies

Ingredients:

1 cup tigernut flour

¾ cup almond flour

¼ cup tapioca flour

¼ cup chopped walnuts

2 tablespoons Hu Chocolate Gems or organic dark chocolate chips

5 teaspoons honey or 5 dates, seeded and diced

1 tablespoon MCT oil

1 tablespoon butter-flavored Nutiva Coconut Oil or extra-virgin coconut oil

1 teaspoon pure vanilla extract

1 tablespoon organic SunButter or other sunflower seed butter

¼ teaspoon salt

¼ teaspoon baking soda

Actions:

1. If you are baking these, preheat the oven to 325°F.

2. Mix all the ingredients in a large bowl until well combined. This should produce a moist dough. Add a splash of water if needed to reach desired consistency. Roll into balls; they are ready to eat!

3. If you are baking the cookies, place the dough balls on a baking tray lined with baking paper. You can also flatten the balls into cookie shapes, if desired.

4. Bake for 7 to 8 minutes, until just golden brown.

Tips:

• If you want to eat the dough raw, roll the balls in cacao powder! It gives a delicious flavor when biting into them.

• For a softer cookie, use blanched almond flour. If you use almond flour that was made with almonds with skins on, you will need to add a little more water.

MINI CASHEW CHEESECAKES

If you love cheesecake, this is the recipe for you. It's a healthy alternative that is free of dairy and refined sugar, and uses cashews instead of cheese! Cashews provide a comforting feeling similar to the one cheese does. Because cashews contain anacardic acids, many studies have been conducted on their anxiolytic effect.[3] One study also proved that daily consumption of cashews reduces oxidative stress.[4]

You'll need paper cupcake liners and a mini cupcake tray for this recipe. (Remember to look for FSC-certified compostable, unbleached, chlorine-free baking cups.)

Total time: 10 minutes to prepare, 40 minutes to set • Makes 20 mini cheesecakes

Ingredients:

3 cups cashew nuts

¾ cup maple syrup

¾ cup coconut oil

½ cup lemon juice

1 tablespoon pure vanilla extract

Pinch of salt

Actions:

1. Soak the cashews in water for 4 hours, then discard the soaking liquid. Put all the ingredients in a high-speed blender and whip until completely smooth. Line a mini cupcake tray with the paper cups.

2. Spoon 1 heaping tablespoon of the mixture into each cupcake cup.

3. Set in the refrigerator for 40 minutes, and they are ready to enjoy!

Tips:

- If you have a very powerful blender, you may be able to skip soaking the cashews.

- Garnish each cupcake with a walnut or pecan to make them even more of a brain food!

- For a different texture, you can let these cheesecakes set in the freezer. They'll set in about 20 minutes.

- If you use a regular-size rather than mini cupcake tin, expect the cheesecakes to take about 80 minutes to set.

CHOCOLATE AVOCADO MOUSSE

This mousse provides an excellent snack or dessert. Enjoy it with some roasted walnuts on top—in fact, always try to think of how you could add more walnuts to your foods, especially desserts! The mousse is super easy to make with just a handful of ingredients.

You can store the mousse in the fridge for up to four days; the honey helps to preserve it.

Total time: 5 minutes • Makes 1 serving

Ingredients:

1 avocado

2 tablespoons cacao powder

2 tablespoons honey

1 teaspoon MCT oil

⅛ teaspoon vanilla extract

Actions:

Blend all the ingredients in a food processor until smooth and creamy. (Alternatively, mash all the ingredients in a bowl with a fork until well combined.)

Tips:

- Serve this mousse garnished with fresh raspberries, strawberries, and walnuts.

- Add a can of coconut cream to yield even more chocolate mousse and add a nice flavor! This will add more health benefits to your mousse, and it will also change its appearance from a dark chocolate to a milk chocolate–colored mousse.

- This mousse makes an excellent frosting for a cake!

CHOCOLATE SAUCE–COVERED STRAWBERRIES

This chocolate sauce is divine! It took me a while to perfect the measurements to get it as creamy and luscious as possible. And then strawberries dipped into it . . . mmm, it is heavenly! This comes out to be more of a fondue than a hard-set chocolate on the strawberries. Nutritionally speaking, this recipe provides magnesium and vitamin C, two nutrients that boost the immune system, relax the body, and reduce anxiety. This is a fun one for kids, too—they love to dip fruit into a delicious chocolate sauce. It's free of dairy and refined sugar, and it's just three ingredients!

Total time: 10 minutes • Makes 1½ cups (6 servings)

Ingredients:

⅔ cup cacao powder
½ cup maple syrup

¼ cup coconut oil, refined
or extra-virgin (see tips)
2 cups organic strawberries

Actions:

1. Add the cacao, maple syrup, and oil to a blender. Mix on high speed until smooth.

2. Dip the strawberries into the sauce and place on a tray. Let set for a few minutes in the freezer or eat right away!

Tips:

- Using a powerful high-speed blender, like the Vitamix, will help whip this chocolate sauce into a thick, smooth texture.

- I like to use Nutiva Coconut Oil, which is refined, for this recipe so it doesn't smell or taste like coconut but has the correct texture and consistency. If you prefer the taste of coconut, you can use extra-virgin coconut oil instead.

- Try dipping other fruits in this chocolate sauce, such as banana and oranges, or even walnuts and macadamia nuts.

- If you want to end up with hard-set chocolate-covered strawberries, you could melt down a healthy chocolate bar, like the ones made by Hu, and then set the strawberries in the fridge after dipping them. This will give you harder chocolate-covered strawberries much like the ones we can buy at the store.

ICE CREAM BITES WITH CHOCOLATE SAUCE

This is one of my all-time favorite recipes, and definitely one of the top 10 recipes I have ever created! These bites are free of dairy and refined sugars. They are so delicious, with the creaminess of the cashews, and the chocolate on top—wow, what a combo! I recommend making these once a week and having them on hand in your freezer, especially if you frequently crave ice cream. They are a great alternative—so much healthier and so nourishing and full of antioxidants. You get the health benefits of the cashews, the cacao, and the coconut oil.

This recipe includes maca, which contains flavonoids that are said to improve mood and reduce anxiety. A 2014 study of postmenopausal women found that maca reduced their feelings of anxiety and depression along with reducing their blood pressure.[5] This is a delicious and nutritious treat to reduce stress.

Total time: 10 minutes preparation, plus soaking and freezing • Makes 15 bites

Ingredients:

1½ cups cashews

½ cup maple syrup

¼ cup coconut oil, refined
  or extra-virgin (see tips)

Juice of 1 small lemon
  (2 to 3 tablespoons)

1 tablespoon vanilla extract

1 teaspoon maca

Dash of salt

1 batch of Chocolate Sauce
  (see p. 250), as a topping

Actions:

1. Soak the cashews in water for 4 hours, then discard the soaking liquid. Blend all the ingredients except the Chocolate Sauce in a blender on high speed until smooth. There should be absolutely no lumps.

2. Scoop this mixture in little mounds onto a parchment-lined baking tray and place in the freezer for 5 minutes.

3. Add a spoonful of Chocolate Sauce to each ice cream bite. Place back in the freezer for 30 minutes and they are ready to enjoy!

Tips:

- If you have a very powerful blender, you may be able to skip soaking the cashews.

- Use a high-powered blender, like the Vitamix, to produce a completely smooth whipped cashew ice cream. There is nothing else like it!

- I like to use Nutiva refined coconut oil for this recipe, because it has been through one more step of refinement than typical extra-virgin coconut oil, so it doesn't taste or smell like coconut, though it provides a perfect, ice cream–like consistency.

CHOCOLATE SUNBUTTER CUPS

These two-ingredient treats come together quickly for a satisfying, yet daringly easy, brain-food snack. All you need are paper baking cups, some dark chocolate bars, and a jar of sunflower seed butter to enjoy these allergy-friendly, better-for-you candies. It doesn't get much easier than this.

Total time: 35 minutes • Makes 12 cups

Ingredients:

2 Hu Dark Chocolate bars, either Salty or Simple, or another organic dark chocolate bar (as long as it has no refined sugar in it)

12 teaspoons organic SunButter or other sunflower seed butter

Actions:

1. Arrange 12 medium-size paper baking cups on a baking sheet.

2. Melt the chocolate bars in a pot over low heat.

3. Drop 1 teaspoon chocolate and 1 teaspoon SunButter into each paper cup. Top the cups with another teaspoon of chocolate, covering the filling completely.

4. Refrigerate for 20 minutes and they're ready to eat!

Tip:

For a great bite-size snack, use mini paper baking cups. They will take 10 to 15 minutes to set, depending on the size of the cups.

CHOCOLATE HAZELNUTELLA

This delicious alternative to the chocolate hazelnut spread that so many people love is free from refined sugar, dairy, and preservatives. Made with a combination of hazelnuts and walnuts, it has a delicious hazelnut flavor, but with a hint of walnut that gives it a divine consistency—along with antioxidants, omega-3s, and anxiolytic effects!

This spread is delicious as a topping on a smoothie bowl or açai bowl, on porridge, or as a dip with fruit. Eat a spoonful for some energy on the go.

Total time: 5 minutes • Makes 1 cup

Ingredients:

¾ cup raw or roasted hazelnuts

¼ cup walnuts

¼ cup honey

¼ cup raw cacao powder

3 tablespoons MCT oil

1 teaspoon vanilla extract

¼ teaspoon sea salt

Action:

Blend all the ingredients in a blender until smooth.

Tip:

You can use a food processor or a blender for this recipe.

PLANT-BASED ICE CREAM

This nondairy ice cream is wonderful served with fresh fruit, nuts, and/or Chocolate Sauce (see p. 250).

Total time: 15 minutes preparation, 3 to 5 hours freezing • Makes 2 servings

Ingredients:

1 cup cashew nuts (substitute sunflower seeds or
   hempseeds if you have nut allergies)

⅔ cup almond milk or tigernut milk

2 dates, seeded

2 tablespoons maple syrup

1 teaspoon vanilla extract

¼ teaspoon salt

Actions:

1. Blend all the ingredients in a food processor or blender until the mixture is as creamy and frothy as you can make it.

2. Pour the mixture into a container and place in the freezer. Allow the ice cream to set in the freezer for 5 hours or overnight.

Tips:

• If you have an ice cream maker, make the recipe in a blender and then pour it into the ice cream maker. Allow to churn for 30 minutes and then it will be ready to eat.

• The more powerful your blender, the creamier your ice cream will be.

• For the creamiest ice cream possible, let the mixture freeze for 1 to 2 hours, or until it's still soft but starting to freeze. Put it back in the blender and blend to a creamy consistency, then return the mixture to the freezer. You can repeat this step one more time if you like!

Variations:

There are many flavors you can make! Try all of these and then invent some of your own.

Chocolate Chip Ice Cream: Add 1 tablespoon cacao powder and 3 tablespoons cacao nibs.

Chocolate Ice Cream: Add 1 tablespoon cacao powder.

Chocolate Mint Ice Cream: Add a handful of mint leaves, a drop of mint extract or food-grade mint essential oil (food grade), and 1 tablespoon cacao powder.

Coffee Ice Cream: Add 1 tablespoon very finely ground espresso.

Cookie Dough Ice Cream: Drop cookie dough into partially frozen ice cream.

Matcha Ice Cream: Add ½ tablespoon matcha (powdered green tea).

Mint Ice Cream: Add a handful of mint leaves and a drop of mint extract.

Strawberry Ice Cream: Add 1 cup strawberries.

Vanilla-Lemon Ice Cream: Add the juice of 1 to 2 lemons.

Vanilla-Lime Ice Cream: Add the juice of 1 to 2 limes.

CHOCOLATE HAZELNUT CAKE

Cake is a classic comfort food! My healthy take on the recipe is dairy-free, gluten-free, and vegan. No refined flours or sugars here!

Total time: 1 hour 10 minutes • Makes 16 servings

Ingredients:

For the cake:

1 cup almond milk or another plant-based milk

1 tablespoon baking soda

1 teaspoon apple cider vinegar

¼ cup flaxseed meal

½ cup plus 2 tablespoons filtered water

3 apples, peeled and cored

⅔ cup coconut sugar

½ cup plus 2 tablespoons maple syrup

1 teaspoon vanilla extract

½ teaspoon salt

½ cup coconut oil, refined or extra-virgin (see tips)

1 cup cacao powder

1½ cups almond flour

1 cup oat flour

½ cup tapioca flour

For the frosting:	*For the topping:*
1½ cups organic powdered sugar	1 cup roasted hazelnuts, chopped
½ cup almond milk	½ cup roasted walnuts, chopped
½ cup cacao powder	
¼ cup maple syrup	
¼ cup butter-flavored Nutiva Coconut Oil (see tips)	

Actions:

1. Preheat the oven to 350°F, and grease an 8-inch round cake pan.

2. Add the almond milk, baking soda, and apple cider vinegar to a large bowl, then stir and let the mixture sit a few minutes to curdle.

3. Add the flax meal and water to a separate bowl. Whisk together well and then set aside. In 5 minutes, the texture will be gummy like eggs.

4. Blend the apples in a food processor until you have applesauce.

5. Add the flax meal mixture, applesauce, coconut sugar, and maple syrup to the almond milk bowl. Whisk well.

6. Add the vanilla, salt, and coconut oil and stir.

7. Whisk together the cacao powder and flours in a separate bowl. Add to the wet mixture, stirring gently.

8. Pour the batter into the cake pan. Bake for 40 to 45 minutes. Let it cool in the tin before removing it from the pan.

9. Make the frosting in a bowl or blender by whipping together all the ingredients until thick and smooth. When the cake is completely cooled, smooth it on.

10. Garnish the outside of the cake with hazelnuts and walnuts and enjoy!

Tips:

- It's easy to make your own oat flour. Simply put oats (like the kind you get for oatmeal) in a blender and process until it's a fine flour consistency.

- In place of the butter-flavored Nutiva Coconut Oil, you can use regular Nutiva Coconut Oil, which is refined, so it doesn't smell or taste like coconut. If you prefer the taste of coconut, you can use extra-virgin coconut oil instead.

GRANOLA PROTEIN BARS WITH CHOCOLATE CHIPS AND SUNBUTTER

Rather than spend a fortune on protein bars that taste kind of blah and have ingredients you don't want, try making these homemade bars. They provide 10 grams of protein per bar, taste delicious, and are full of superfoods for the brain! The chocolate chips are sweetened with coconut sugar, rather than cane sugar, and are free of dairy, soy, and other additives. This is a no-bake recipe, making it as simple as adding the ingredients to a bowl and mixing. These bars are made up of all kinds of antianxiety superfoods, including roasted sunflower seed butter, walnuts, oats, chia seeds, hempseeds, cacao, and coconut oil.

Total time: 10 minutes • Makes 21 bars

Ingredients:

1½ cups organic SunButter or other sunflower seed butter

1 cup oats

1 cup Hu Chocolate Gems or cacao nibs

½ cup tigernut flour or almond flour

⅓ cup walnuts, chopped

5 dates, seeded and chopped

¼ cup chia seeds

¼ cup hempseeds

2 tablespoons honey

1 tablespoon coconut oil

1 tablespoon MCT oil

¼ teaspoon vanilla extract

¼ teaspoon sea salt

Actions:

1. Mix all the ingredients in a bowl until they are moist enough to stick together.

2. Pat the mixture into a 9 x 13-inch glass baking dish, let set in the fridge for 60 minutes, and then cut into bars.

FRUIT LEATHERS

I put this recipe in the book for candy lovers! You can satisfy your cravings and feel fulfilled as a cook in the process by making homemade Fruit Leathers. Each one takes less than 10 minutes of hands-on time to prepare, but they do need to be dehydrated for a few hours. Cherry Fruit Leather is my favorite!

Note: If you love these, I recommend getting a food dehydrator, as having the oven on for this amount of time may not be ideal—unless, of course, it's winter!

Actions:

1. Add the fruits of your choice to a food processor, and blend until smooth.

2. *Dehydrator method:* Place parchment paper on the mesh screens in your dehydrator. Pour the fruit mixture on the paper, and smooth to an even, ¼-inch-thick layer. Dehydrate at 115°F for 8 to 12 hours, or until no longer wet.

3. *Oven method:* Pour the mixture onto a large baking tray lined with a silicone sheet or parchment paper for easier cleanup. Smooth it out to an even, ¼-inch-thick layer. Bake in your preheated oven at 150°F for 4 to 6 hours, until it is sticky and sweet like candy.

Here are some variations:

CHERRY LEATHER

Ingredient:
8 cups cherries, seeded

STRAWBERRY KIWIFRUIT LEATHER

Ingredients:
2 cups strawberries, destemmed
10 kiwifruit, peeled

PLUM LEATHER

Ingredient:
8 cups plums, seeded

STRAWBERRY APPLE LEATHER

Ingredients:
2 cups strawberries
4 apples, cored and peeled

PEACH APPLE LEATHER

Ingredients:
4 apples, cored and peeled
4 peaches, seeded

APRICOT LEATHER

Ingredient:
8 cups fresh apricots, seeded

ELDERBERRY GUMMY BEARS

Elderberry is a powerful immune system booster. Boosting our immune system is one way to reduce anxiety. You will need gummy molds (bear-shaped or not!) in which to set the gummy bear mixture and a medicine dropper to fill them. Be sure to get some that are BPA-free.

Total time: 15 minutes • Makes 50 gummies

Ingredients:

2 to 3 tablespoons coconut oil to grease the molds

1 cup elderberry syrup

½ cup filtered water

½ tablespoon agar powder or gelatin

2 tablespoons honey

Actions:

1. Place some coconut oil on a paper towel and grease the gummy molds lightly.

2. Combine the elderberry syrup, water, and agar powder in a pot and bring to a boil; reduce the heat to low and let simmer for 5 minutes.

3. Stir continuously until the agar is completely dissolved. Remove from the heat and mix in the honey.

4. Use the medicine dropper to fill the gummy molds with the elderberry mixture.

5. Refrigerate for 3 hours until completely set. Keep in a jar in the fridge and eat within 60 days.

CHOCOLATE-DIPPED ORANGES
WITH ROASTED HAZELNUTS AND WALNUTS

These treats are a combination of cacao and citrus, a powerful duo in boosting the immune system and reducing anxiety!

Total time: 40 minutes • Makes 14 pieces

Ingredients:

½ cup hazelnuts

½ cup walnuts

2 Hu Dark Chocolate bars, either Salty or Simple, or another organic dark chocolate bar

2 oranges or 4 tangerines, peeled and separated

Actions:

1. Preheat the oven to 350°F.

2. Chop the hazelnuts and walnuts into small pieces in a food processor. Spread the nuts over a baking tray and roast for 3 to 5 minutes, watching carefully to be sure the nuts don't burn.

3. Melt the chocolate bars in a small pot over low heat.

4. Dip the citrus wedges into the melted chocolate, then into the roasted nuts until they are well covered. Arrange the fruit on a baking tray lined with parchment paper. Refrigerate for 20 minutes.

MOIST CHOCOLATE SUNBUTTER BROWNIES

These no-bake brownies are so moist and delicious! They are free of gluten, dairy, and refined sugar. Roasted sunflower seed butter makes the brownies truly nourishing, as sunflowers came in at #3 of all the nuts and seeds on the Antioxidant Food Table.

Total time: 20 minutes • Makes 24 brownies

Ingredients:

For the brownies:

1½ cups plus 2 tablespoons tigernut flour or almond flour

1 cup organic SunButter or other sunflower seed butter

1 cup cacao powder

¾ cup maple syrup

5 tablespoons filtered water

1 teaspoon vanilla extract

Dash of sea salt

For the topping:

¼ cup organic SunButter or other sunflower seed butter

½ cup Hu Chocolate Gems or cacao nibs

Actions:

1. Add all the brownie ingredients to a bowl. Mix until well combined.
2. Press the brownie mixture into a baking tray lined with parchment paper.
3. Smooth a layer of SunButter on top of the brownies.
4. Sprinkle the chocolate gems over the SunButter.
5. Put in the refrigerator for 1 hour to set, then cut into 24 squares. They're ready to eat and enjoy!

CHOCOLATE SUNBUTTER SPREAD

This is the easiest homemade spread ever, and it has a unique, delicious flavor. The combo of chocolate and sunflower seed butter is the ultimate anxiety reducer.

Have a spoonful for a burst of energy before a workout or when you're on the go. This is also lovely paired with fruit such as apple, apricot, or banana slices, or as a topping on an açai bowl, smoothie bowl, or oats.

Total time: 5 minutes • Makes 1⅓ cups

Ingredients:

1 cup organic SunButter

3 tablespoons cacao

2 tablespoons honey

Actions:

Add all the ingredients to a jar and stir until combined; it's ready to eat! Refrigerate in the jar. The spread will keep for 60 days—if you can restrain yourself from eating it all right away!

Tip:

If you can't source a sunflower seed butter, blend sunflower seeds in your food processor until you achieve your desired consistency.

CHAPTER 14

Seven-Day Guide for Living Anxiety-Free

Follow this plan as best you can. If you can adhere to it 100 percent that would be ideal; however, even if you don't follow it to the letter, it's likely that by eating this way on some of the days you will still be consuming more omega fats and antioxidants in a week than you would ordinarily. Always remember, especially with anxiety, that making *some* effort to feel better is better than doing nothing.

Over the next seven days, pay attention to how you feel while you are eating. Then check again to see how you feel 30 minutes later, an hour later, and the next day. This will be a good awareness exercise for you. You may want to keep a journal or notes in your phone to track your moods along with your food.

Many people report improvement in as little as a week once they begin deliberately nourishing their nervous system. For the most part, you can expect to feel an increase of energy and a sense of calmness because you are nourishing your gut, brain, and nervous system with proven antianxiety foods, including plenty of fruits and vegetables that are sources of antioxidants, anti-inflammatories, B vitamins, and omega-3s, and eggs, fish, nuts, and other foods rich in amino acids (tryptophan, tyrosine, phenylalanine) that are the precursors of dopamine.

Over the next week, you will be helping the cells in your gut release serotonin, the so-called happy hormone, so I hope you feel more at ease.

Over the first few days, it is possible that you could experience some minor detox symptoms—slight achiness, fatigue, irritability, sadness, diarrhea, or insomnia have been reported by some people when they first clean up their eating habits. These symptoms should be mild and pass within a day or two. If you get any of these, boost your water consumption a bit. Rest. Let your body heal.

If you have any questions at all, please contact me through my website www.LianaWernerGray.com. I also encourage you to post pictures of your meals and tag me on Instagram: @theearthdiet.

It is going to be a great week.

Caution: If you have digestive issues or any medical issues, or are on medication for any condition, it's a good idea to check in with your doctor before beginning. You'll want to make sure that the ingredients are fine for your condition and that nothing (such as St. John's wort) will affect any medications you are taking.

Work with a doctor you trust and make sure your doctor has some nutritional knowledge. Bear in mind that most doctors are not nutritional experts, so you may need to find a specialist. It's important to have someone who believes in offering holistic care, including nutritional solutions, alongside any necessary medication.

General Notes

The same recipes are alternated at intervals throughout the week, making meal prep as easy as possible. Vegans should swap plant-based meals for meat-eater meals, wherever those appear, and be sure to take a daily B-complex vitamin supplement.

Feel free to repeat the menus in this guide for as many weeks as you like. I have made this plan the foundation of my personal diet because we can get all the nutrients we need from following it.

Here is an overview of the daily plan.

- Upon rising: Lemon Chlorophyll Water (p. 168) and supplements
- Breakfast
- Snack
- Lunch
- Snack
- Dinner
- Dessert (optional)
- Tea before bed

Breakfast options include:

- Brainiac Porridge (p. 175)
- Omelet (p. 182)
- Genius Smoothie (p. 158)
- Brain Bowl (p. 179)

Lunch and dinner options include:

- Baked Walnut-Crusted Salmon (p. 234)
- Walnut-Crusted Chicken (p. 236)
- Superfood Kale Salad (vegan) (p. 212)
- Broccoli Popcorn (vegan) (p. 190)
- Grass-Fed Beef Burrito (p. 230)

- Creamy, Delicious GF Mac 'n' Cheese (vegan) (p. 191)

- Green Sprout Salad (vegan) (p. 210)

- Cauliflower-Cheese Pesto Lasagna (vegan) (p. 197)

If you want to switch out any of these meals, you can. Pick anything from Part II, "Anxiety-Free with Food Recipes." A good alternate for those who consume meat would be Baked Fish with Yucca (p. 238). A good alternate for vegans (and also meat eaters) would be Grounding Lentil Soup with Avocado and Ginger (p. 205).

Snack and dessert options include fresh juices. These have so many benefits for soothing the nervous system that it is important to have at least one of these every day.

- Super Greens Juice (p. 153)

- Beet Juice (p. 154)

- Hotshot Citrus (p. 160)

The best snacks are always ingredients in their natural state, such as a raw vegetable, a piece of fruit, or a handful of nuts and/ or seeds. I have included these snacks in your plan for the next seven days. For these options you also can choose from among the dessert recipes listed below. These may help alleviate anxiety because of the high antioxidant content, especially the Genius Chocolate Balls. You can, at any time, of course, replace a chocolate ball with an orange or apple.

If you enjoy one dessert in particular, make a batch and it will last you the entire week. If you usually eat a lot of ice cream, chocolate, and cookies, I recommend making all of the recipes below, so you'll have enough on hand whenever a craving strikes. This way you'll be assured that you're getting excellent nutrition while satisfying the craving.

- Ice Cream Bites with Chocolate Sauce (p. 251)

- Chocolate Sauce–Covered Strawberries (p. 250)

- Smart Cookies (p. 247)
- Genius Chocolate Balls (p. 246)

Tea is to be had at bedtime to cap off the day, in a way, as well as to help you relax for a good night's sleep. However, you can drink as much noncaffeinated tea as you like throughout the day. Make sure it includes one of these ingredients:

- St. John's wort (p. 97)
- Lemon balm (p. 89)
- Rhodiola (p. 96)
- Ginger (p. 53)

I recommend picking Sunday to be your prep day and Monday to be your start day. But if you're eager to get started right away, pick any day you want to begin! The following plan is designed to serve one individual; however, if you make the Walnut-Crusted Chicken recipe, for example, which could serve four people at one sitting, you can eat it for dinner and then have the other portions as leftovers.

If this plan includes too much food for you, keep your portions small and skip a meal or a snack here and there. Just keep in mind that skipping too many meals is counterproductive. The purpose of this plan is to provide an abundance of nourishment to your brain and body in the form of nutrients that are recognized as being supportive for anxiety. Among other things, these nutrients will help restore your adrenal glands and calm your nervous system. Soothing anxiety is not about counting calories or macros, it's about taking all that good stuff in.

Following this plan will ensure that you are having a green drink daily by starting with Lemon Water with Chlorophyll and your supplements. I recommend that vegans take B-complex and that everyone take a daily support (such as two of my Anxiety-Free supplements) at this time. Then you will also getting liquid nutrition from alternating between a smoothie, green juice, and beet juice each day.

SUNDAY—PREP DAY

Planning for success has only two steps, but it can take a few hours.

1. Go shopping for all the ingredients you need. I like to order online because it's convenient and even budget-friendly; I compare prices with sales and am not so tempted to purchase things that aren't on my list. If you place an order for delivery, make sure to order what you need a week before starting, so you have all your ingredients ready to go. (If you order online for pickup or same-day delivery, your timing needs may vary.)

2. Make all your desserts for the week ahead.

7-DAY MEAL PLAN

MONDAY—DAY 1

Upon rising: Lemon Water with Chlorophyll and supplements

Breakfast: Brainiac Porridge

Snack: Super Greens Juice

Lunch: Superfood Kale Salad

Snack: An orange

Dinner: Walnut-Crusted Chicken Salad
(save some for lunch on Day 2)

Dessert (optional): Anything from the choices
on hand or a piece of fruit

Before bedtime: St. John's Wort Tea

TUESDAY—DAY 2

Upon rising: Lemon Water with Chlorophyll and supplements

Breakfast: Genius Smoothie

Snack: Genius Chocolate Balls

Lunch: Walnut-Crusted Chicken Salad

Snack: Beet Juice

Dinner: Creamy, Delicious Vegan GF Mac 'n' Cheese
(save some for lunch on Day 3)

Dessert (optional): Anything from the choices on hand or a
piece of fruit

Before bedtime: St. John's Wort Tea

WEDNESDAY—DAY 3

Upon rising: Lemon Water with Chlorophyll and supplements

Breakfast: Omelet

Snack: Citrus Smoothie

Lunch: Creamy, Delicious Vegan GF Mac 'n' Cheese

Snack: Cashew Ice Cream Bites with Chocolate Sauce

Dinner: Baked Walnut-Crusted Salmon
(save some for lunch on Day 4)

Dessert (optional): Anything from the choices
on hand or a piece of fruit

Before bedtime: Lemon Balm Tea

THURSDAY—DAY 4

Upon rising: Lemon Water with Chlorophyll and supplements

Breakfast: Brainiac Porridge

Snack: Super Greens Juice

Lunch: Walnut-Crusted Salmon

Snack: Chocolate Sauce–Covered Strawberries

Dinner: Superfood Kale Salad with Broccoli Popcorn

Dessert (optional): Anything from the choices
on hand or a piece of fruit

Before bedtime: Ginger Tea

FRIDAY—DAY 5

Upon rising: Lemon Water with Chlorophyll and supplements

Breakfast: Genius Smoothie

Snack: Beet Juice

Lunch: Green Sprout Salad

Snack: Cookie Dough

Dinner: Grass-Fed Beef Burrito (save some for lunch on Day 6)

Dessert (optional): Anything from the choices on hand or a
piece of fruit

Before bedtime: Ginger Tea

SATURDAY—DAY 6

Upon rising: Lemon Water with Chlorophyll and supplements

Breakfast: Omelet

Snack: Citrus Smoothie

Lunch: Grass-Fed Beef Burrito

Snack: Genius Chocolate Balls

Dinner: Cauliflower-Cheese Pesto Lasagna
(save some for lunch on Day 7)

Dessert (optional): Anything from the choices
on hand or a piece of fruit

Before bedtime: Rhodiola Tea

SUNDAY—DAY 7

Upon rising: Lemon Water with Chlorophyll and supplements

Breakfast: Brain Bowl

Snack: Super Greens Juice

Lunch: Cauliflower-Cheese Pesto Lasagna

Snack: Cashew Ice Cream Bites with Chocolate Sauce

Dinner: Green Sprout Salad

Dessert (optional): Anything from the choices
on hand or a piece of fruit

Before bedtime: Rhodiola Tea

Just Do Your Best and Know I'm on Your Side

Come to my website (www.LianaWernerGray.com/AnxietyFree) to download a free checklist of the Seven-Day Plan. Personally, I find I get a sense of accomplishment when committing to a week like this. I love to tick the box every time I have a Lemon Water with some chlorophyll or eat a nutritionally supportive meal. Psychologists say that goal setting and achievement are very positive for people experiencing anxiety, and I agree.

That said, I encourage you to strive for progress, not perfection. Even if you start the plan and don't finish it or do 50 percent, be happy for yourself. That would be amazing. I don't care about anything other than seeing you practice self-care so you can gain some relief and be happy. Remember this: You played ball on the court. You were in action. This is the most important thing.

Let's focus on the positives, as we don't need any negative thoughts firing off and generating more anxious chemistry in our bodies!

Stick to the guidelines to create an anxiety-free body, an environment in which anxiety has no residence and is not supported or sustained. Let's make our brains, guts, and nervous systems impervious to anxiety and resilient to whatever life throws at us.

METRIC CONVERSION CHART

Standard Cup	Fine Powder (e.g., flour)	Grain (e.g., rice)	Granular (e.g., sugar)	Liquid Solids (e.g., butter)	Liquid (e.g., milk)
1	140 g	150 g	190 g	200 g	240 ml
¾	105 g	113 g	143 g	150 g	180 ml
⅔	93 g	100 g	125 g	133 g	160 ml
½	70 g	75 g	95 g	100 g	120 ml
⅓	47 g	50 g	63 g	67 g	80 ml
¼	35 g	38 g	48 g	50 g	60 ml
⅛	18 g	19 g	24 g	25 g	30 ml

Useful Equivalents for Liquid Ingredients by Volume				
¼ tsp			1 ml	
½ tsp			2 ml	
1 tsp			5 ml	
3 tsp	1 tbsp		½ fl oz	15 ml
	2 tbsp	⅛ cup	1 fl oz	30 ml
	4 tbsp	¼ cup	2 fl oz	60 ml
	5⅓ tbsp	⅓ cup	3 fl oz	80 ml
	8 tbsp	½ cup	4 fl oz	120 ml
	10⅔ tbsp	⅔ cup	5 fl oz	160 ml
	12 tbsp	¾ cup	6 fl oz	180 ml
	16 tbsp	1 cup	8 fl oz	240 ml
	1 pt	2 cups	16 fl oz	480 ml
	1 qt	4 cups	32 fl oz	960 ml
			33 fl oz	1000 ml	1 L

Useful Equivalents for Dry Ingredients by Weight		
(To convert ounces to grams, multiply the number of ounces by 30.)		
1 oz	1/16 lb	30 g
4 oz	1/4 lb	120 g
8 oz	1/2 lb	240 g
12 oz	3/4 lb	360 g
16 oz	1 lb	480 g

Useful Equivalents for Cooking/Oven Temperatures			
Process	Fahrenheit	Celsius	Gas Mark
Freeze Water	32° F	0° C	
Room Temperature	68° F	20° C	
Boil Water	212° F	100° C	
Bake	325° F	160° C	3
	350° F	180° C	4
	375° F	190° C	5
	400° F	200° C	6
	425° F	220° C	7
	450° F	230° C	8
Broil			Grill

Useful Equivalents for Length				
(To convert inches to centimeters, multiply the number of inches by 2.5.)				
1 in			2.5 cm	
6 in	1/2 ft		15 cm	
12 in	1 ft		30 cm	
36 in	3 ft	1 yd	90 cm	
40 in			100 cm	1 m

RESOURCES

Visit my website, LianaWernerGray.com, for discount codes on products, for ongoing support and information, for news of events across the United States and around the world, to join my newsletter, and to link to my activity on various social networks. That's the hub of my world. Connect with me there anytime.

Here, you will find resources that are helpful in achieving overall health and well-being, as well as in reducing anxiety. These are all things that I personally have in my home or use on a regular basis, and for good reason.

RESOURCES FOR THE KITCHEN

Organic non-GMO food brands I use in my recipes:

- *SunButter roasted sunflower seed butter:* I use the certified organic one (there are a few to choose from) with just one ingredient, roasted sunflower seeds.

- *Nutiva:* My brand of choice for coconut oil, avocado oil, MCT oil, protein powder, hempseeds, chia seeds, and coconut sugar.

- *Hu:* This company makes organic chocolate that is dairy-free and sweetened with coconut sugar. There are no fillers or additives in it, just simple ingredients like cacao powder, cacao butter, and coconut sugar flavored with nuts, mint, sea salt, or quinoa.

- *Explore Cuisine:* This company makes gluten-free pastas from beans that are out of this world—red lentil penne, edamame mung bean fettuccini, black bean spaghetti, chickpea spaghetti, green lentil lasagna—and chickpea rice (*risoni!*).

- *Stockton Aloe 1:* We want pure aloe with absolutely no preservatives or anything else added. Aloe juice sold in supermarkets and organic stores typically contains some preservative to make it shelf-stable. But this brand does not have any preservatives. This product is frozen when it's fresh and gets shipped on dry ice. Its freshness is what makes it so nutritionally potent! Just like fresh apples beat canned apples for nutritional value, fresh aloe beats preserved aloe. Use this link for a discount and to receive a free gift of an aloe lotion: https://aloe1.com/shop/aloe-1-58-oz -incl-aloe-cream/?ref=56 .

- *Ancient Nutrition:* This is my source for bone broth and collagen. The company was founded by chiropractor and nutritionist Dr. Josh Axe and natural health expert Jordan Rubin.

For a downloadable "Anxiety-Free Ingredients" shopping list and online discount codes for ordering all the products I recommend, visit LianaWernerGray.com/AnxietyFree. (Don't pay full price if you don't need to!)

Appliances

- *Vitamix blenders:* The most efficient high-speed blender line on the market! A Vitamix will whip cashews so smooth to make creamy cream, ice cream, and cheesecake. You can make delicious smoothies, sauces, and even soups in one of these.

- *Nama Vitality 5800 cold-press juicer:* This juice machine makes cold-pressed juices, as well as smoothies and nut milks! It has a patented technology that enables us to extract more juice and vital micronutrients from fruits and vegetables, compared to the fast juice machines that zap the fruits and vegetables with a blade and don't extract as much juice as possible. Use the code LIANA for 10 percent off at NamaWell.com.

- *Echo water filter:* I use the Echo, which is a hydrogen filter. Over the past 11 years, I researched, tried, and experimented with different water filters. This was my favorite and is now the one I have in my apartment. Also please note, no company could pay me enough to say their product is the "best." I simply want to personally use the best one in my home, so it has to be the most effective to support this healthy life. The filter removes chlorine and fluoride, and alkalizes and adds hydrogen to water.

  Hydrogen is the crucial piece of this technology to understand. The hydrogen in this filter is a miracle, as water is simply the very best delivery mechanism to get hydrogen where it needs to go, which is into the gut, in the most bioavailable form possible. As you know, if you have anxiety, your gut may be in trouble. Everyone's gut is designed—when functioning properly—to produce up to eight liters of hydrogen per day. The problem is that the gut is only capable of doing that if it is being fed fresh, raw, organic produce as its main source of fuel. Getting our hydrogen from another source is therefore critical until we can restore the gut to its proper state. Hydrogen is a strategic nutrient to win the fight against inflammation and oxidative stress. Hydrogen also helps to boost brain activity.

  Get more details on the Echo at LianasWater.com.

RESOURCES FOR SKIN CARE

Visit LianaWernerGray.com/AnxietyFree for recommended skin care products. We are not only what we eat but also what we put on our skin. After all, our skin is the largest organ and absorbs what we feed it. Do we want to feed it lotions and toxic ingredients that get absorbed into the blood stream and affect the brain and nervous system?

RESOURCES FOR RETRAINING THE CONSCIOUS MIND

AM-QEC: Our belief systems dictate our perceptions about the world we live in. These then determine the way we internalize and experience that reality. The conscious mind (the part of our mind which we are aware of) processes 2,000 bits of information per second. However, our subconscious mind (which runs everything in the background without our awareness) processes 4 million bits of information per second. The subconscious controls 95 percent or more of our reality. For effective and lasting change to occur, the belief systems dictating our reality, which lie in our subconscious, must first be changed.

AM-QEC is a powerful method by which we can effectively upgrade the "software" of our minds, similar to upgrading a computer system. Originally developed by Melanie Salmon and then refined by Dr. Rashid A. Buttar, AM-QEC essentially allows us to access and efficiently rewire our subconscious belief systems, resulting in significant and lasting change in our lives.

To sign up, go to AdvancedMedicine.com and enter my invitation code: 18737.

RESOURCES FOR CLEAN AIR

Intellipure air purifier: When I first started the Earth Diet, I knew that the end goal would be to make my overall lifestyle as natural and healthy as possible. It started with food, then skin care and household products, and now it's changing my environment to be as natural as possible, which can be a challenge in today's world, as we face polluted air and contaminated water. There is technology that can help us, like air and water purifiers. These are two sound investments, and studies have shown how breathing in the air that most people inhale is quite toxic and causing many health issues.

The statistics are shocking. The World Health Organization (WHO) estimates that 9 of every 10 people worldwide inhale polluted air, and exposure to polluted air is accountable for 7 million deaths annually. I did not know that so many people were dying each year from polluted air! Did you? And it's not a small number, either!

The thing about our air is, we breathe it in all day every day, obviously; however, we don't *see* what we are breathing in. There is particulate matter floating around in the air, and although we can't see it, we can actually buy an air tester and test the air wherever we are. If the air reads zero, that means there is no particulate matter in the air at all, but this just does not happen unless you have an air purifier.

I tested the air in my apartment in New York City, and it wasn't bad, it was 500,000, which may sound like a lot, but some people's apartments are 1.2 million. If it's over 600,000, we should not be breathing that air in if we can avoid it. Rest assured, now I have an air purifier, so I am breathing the cleanest air possible.

So, what is the particulate matter made up of? It could be dust, mold, hair, and even viruses—things we do not want to breathe in. This toxic particulate matter has been proven to cause oxidative stress on the body, and evidence shows us that it is extremely neurotoxic and leads to anxiety and depression. Do we wonder why so many people have anxiety and depression? With the air we breathe and food we eat, no wonder our brains are a toxic mess. Air pollutants can adversely affect our minds and moods. Breathing toxic air leads to respiratory issues, and respiratory issues can cause anxiety because difficulty getting air triggers a fight-or-flight response in the body.

When the COVID-19 pandemic broke out, many hospitals around the world ordered the Intellipure air filter and started using it immediately. Some hospitals put one by every patient's bed. It is my wish that every household in the world would have an air purifier; it is just something that we need in a time like this. These companies provide payment plans, so it makes it affordable for all of us.

Go to www.intellipure.com and enter code LIANA for 10 percent off your purchase.

ANXIETY-FREE DAILY SUPPORT SUPPLEMENTS

The Anxiety-Free supplements that were inspired by the writing of this book are now available. While doing the research, I yearned for an all-organic formula of the most powerful supplements I was discovering, including ashwagandha, spirulina, turmeric, flax seed, chlorella, and schisandra . . . so I went out and made one! I tested the formula on myself, and within days I noticed a major improvement in my ability to focus, my nervous system was calmer, my anxiety was reduced, and I felt more able to effectively deal with stress. All the ingredients are organic and not only boost your immunity but also your levels of important calming neurotransmitters. I am so excited for you to try them, especially with the Seven-Day Guide in Chapter 14!

Visit LianaWernergray.com/AnxietyFreeSupps for more information, including where to purchase them.

ENDNOTES

Introduction

1. S.E. Lakhan and K.F. Vieira, "The Ethical Ramifications of Biomarker Use for Mood Disorders," chap. 18 in *Handbook of Schizophrenia Spectrum Disorders, Volume III: Therapeutic Approaches, Comorbidity, and Outcomes*, ed. M.S. Ritsner (New York: Springer, 2011), doi: 10.1007/978-94-007-0834-1_18.

2. "Mental Health Disorder Statistics," Johns Hopkins Medicine (accessed May 18, 2020), https://www.hopkinsmedicine.org/health/wellness-and -prevention/mental-health-disorder-statistics.

3. J.K. Kiecolt-Glaser et al., "Omega-3 Supplementation Lowers Inflammation and Anxiety in Medical Students: A Randomized Controlled Trial," *Brain, Behavior, and Immunity*, vol. 25, no. 8 (November 2011): 1725–34, doi: 10.1016/j.bbi.2011.07.229.

4. Health Library, University of Michigan (accessed May 18, 2020), https://www.uofmhealth.org/health-library.

5. J.C. Felger. "Imaging the Role of Inflammation in Mood and Anxiety-related Disorders," *Current Neuropharmacology*, vol. 16, no. 5 (June 2018): 533–58, doi: 10.2174/1570159X15666171123201142.

Chapter 1

1. "What Is Stress?" American Institute of Stress (accessed May 11, 2020), https://www.stress.org/what-is-stress.

2. R.M. Hirschfeld, "The Comorbidity of Major Depression and Anxiety Disorders: Recognition and Management in Primary Care," *Primary Care Companion to the Journal of Clinical Psychiatry*, vol. 3, no. 6 (December 2001): 244–54, doi: 10.4088/pcc.v03n0609.

3. K.M. Davison and B.J. Kaplan, "Food Intake and Blood Cholesterol Levels of Community-Based Adults with Mood Disorders," *BMC Psychiatry*, vol. 12, no. 1 (February 2012): 10, doi: 10.1186/1471-244X-12-10.

4. Q. Huang et al., "Linking What We Eat to Our Mood: A Review of Diet, Dietary Antioxidants, and Depression," *Antioxidants*, vol. 8, no. 9 (September 2019): 376, doi: 10.3390/antiox8090376.

5. M. Aucoin and S. Bhardwaj, "Generalized Anxiety Disorder and Hypoglycemia Symptoms Improved with Diet Modification," *Case Reports in Psychiatry,* vol. 2016 (2016): 7165425, doi: 10.1155/2016/7165425.

6. A. Basu et al., "Effects of Dietary Strawberry Supplementation on Antioxidant Biomarkers in Obese Adults with Above Optimal Serum Lipids," *Journal of Nutrition and Metabolism,* vol. 2016 (2016): 3910630, doi: 10.1155/2016/3910630.

7. M. Teychenne, S.A. Costigan, and K. Parker, "The Association between Sedentary Behaviour and Risk of Anxiety: A Systematic Review," *BMC Public Health*, vol. 15 (2015): 513, doi: 10.1186/s12889-015-1843-x; M.F. Masana et al., "Dietary Patterns and Their Association with Anxiety Symptoms among Older Adults: The ATTICA Study," *Nutrients,* vol. 11, no. 6 (June 2019): 1250, doi: 10.3390/nu11061250.

8. M.G. Kutlu and T.J. Gould, "Nicotine Modulation of Fear Memories and Anxiety: Implications for Learning and Anxiety Disorders," *Biochem Pharmacol*, vol. 97, no. 4 (2015): 498–511, doi:10.1016/j.bcp.2015.07.029.

9. "What's in a Cigarette?" American Lung Association (accessed May 18, 2020), https://www.lung.org/quit-smoking/smoking-facts/whats-in-a-cigarette.

10. A. Ströhle and F. Holsboer, "Stress Responsive Neurohormones in Depression and Anxiety," *Pharmacopsychiatry*, vol. 36, supp. 3 (November 2003): s207–14, doi: 10.1055/s-2003-45132.

11. J. Bouayed, H. Rammal, and R. Soulimani, "Oxidative Stress and Anxiety: Relationship and Cellular Pathways," *Oxidative Medicine and Cellular Longevity*, vol. 2, no. 2 (April–June 2009): 63–7, doi: 10.4161/oxim.2.2.7944.

12. F. Ng et al., "Oxidative Stress in Psychiatric Disorders: Evidence Base and Therapeutic Implications," *International Journal of Neuropsychopharmacology*, vol. 11, no. 6 (September 2008): 851–76, doi: 10.1017/S1461145707008401.

13. C.M. Phillips et al., "Dietary Inflammatory Index and Mental Health: A Cross-Sectional Analysis of the Relationship with Depressive Symptoms, Anxiety and Well-Being in Adults," *Journal of Clinical Nutrition*, vol. 37, no. 5 (October 2018): 1485-91, doi: 10.1016/j.clnu.2017.08.029; F. Saghafian et al., "Consumption of Fruit and Vegetables in Relation with Psychological Disorders in Iranian Adults," *European Journal of Nutrition*, vol. 57, no. 6 (September 2018): 2295-2306, doi: 10.1007/s00394-018-1652-y.

14. E. Biringer et al., "The Association Between Depression, Anxiety, and Cognitive Function in the Elderly General Population: The Hordaland Health Study," *International Journal of Geriatric Psychiatry*, vol. 20, no. 10 (October 2005): 989–97, doi: 10.1002/gps.1390.

15. A. Bendix, "8 Signs Your Intermittent Fasting Diet Has Become Unsafe or Unhealthy," *Business Insider* (July 26, 2019)(accessed April 22, 2020), https://www.businessinsider.com/signs-intermittent-fasting-unsafe-unhealthy-2019-7.

16. R. Balon, "Mood, Anxiety, and Physical Illness: Body and Mind, or Mind and Body?" *Depression and Anxiety*, vol. 23, no. 6 (2006): 377–87, doi: 10.1002/da.20217.

17. Janet L. Cummings, "Why Do Anti-Anxiety Medications Sometimes Increase Anxiety?" Cummings Graduate Institute for Behavioral Health Studies, https://cgi.edu/news/anti-anxiety-medications-sometimes-increase-anxiety.

18. Anil Nischal et al., "Suicide and Antidepressants: What Current Evidence Indicates," *Mens Sana Monographs*, vol. 10, no. 1 (Jan-Dec 2012): 33–44, doi: 10.4103/0973-1229.87287.

19. R.F.M. Silva and L. Pogačnik, "Food, Polyphenols and Neuroprotection," *Neural Regeneration Research*, vol. 12, no. 4 (April 2017): 582–3, doi: 10.4103/1673-5374.205096.

20. F.P. Martin et al., "Metabolic Effects of Dark Chocolate Consumption on Energy, Gut Microbiota, and Stress-Related Metabolism in Free-Living Subjects," *Journal of Proteome Research*, vol. 8, no. 12 (December 2009): 5568–79, doi: 10.1021/pr900607v.

21. T.A. Jenkins et al., "Influence of Tryptophan and Serotonin on Mood and Cognition with a Possible Role of the Gut-Brain Axis," *Nutrients*, vol. 8, no. 1 (January 20, 2016): 56, doi: 10.3390/nu8010056.

22. S. Thomas et al., "The Host Microbiome Regulates and Maintains Human Health: A Primer and Perspective for Non-Microbiologists," *Cancer Research*, vol. 77, no. 8 (March 14, 2017): 1783–1812, doi: 10.1158/0008-5472. CAN-16-2929.

23. J. Stoller-Conrad, "Microbes Help Produce Serotonin in Gut," Caltech University (April 9, 2015), https://www.caltech.edu/about/news/microbes-help-produce-serotonin-gut-46495.

24. E. Selhub, "Nutritional Psychiatry: Your Brain on Food," *Harvard Health Blog* (November 16, 2015, updated March 26, 2020), https://www.health.harvard.edu/blog/nutritional-psychiatry-your-brain-on-food-201511168626.

25. "Not All Milk Is Created Equal," Redmond Heritage Farms (accessed April 10, 2020), https://www.redmondfarms.com/milkdifference.

26. B. Yang et al., "Effects of Regulating Intestinal Microbiota on Anxiety Symptoms: A Systematic Review," *General Psychiatry*, vol. 32, no. 2 (May 17, 2019): e100056, doi: 10.1136/gpsych-2019-100056.

27. J.G. Millichap and M.M. Yee, "The Diet Factor in Attention-Deficit/Hyperactivity Disorder," *Pediatrics*, vol. 129, no. 9 (February 2012): 330–7, doi: 10.1542/peds.2011-2199.

28. Kaitlyn Oliphant and Emma Allen-Vercoe, "Macronutrient Metabolism by the Human Gut Microbiome: Major Fermentation By-products and Their Impact on Host Health," *Microbiome*, vol. 7, no. 1 (June 13, 2019): 91, doi:10.1186/s40168-019-0704-8

29. R.P. Mensink and M.B. Katan, "An Epidemiological and an Experimental Study on the Effect of Olive Oil on Total Serum and HDL Cholesterol in Healthy Volunteers," *European Journal of Clinical Nutrition*, vol. 43, supp. 2 (1989): 43–8, PMID: 2557203.

30. "Dopamine," *Psychology Today* (accessed April 17, 2020), https://www. psychologytoday.com/us/basics/dopamine.

31. M. Briguglio et al., "Dietary Neurotransmitters: A Narrative Review on Current Knowledge," *Nutrients*, vol. 10, no. 5 (May 13, 2018): 591, doi: 10.3390/nu10050591.

32. M.J. Breus, "3 Amazing Benefits of GABA," *Psychology Today* (January 3, 2019), https://www.psychologytoday.com/us/blog/ sleep-newzzz/201901/3-amazing-benefits-gaba.

33. N. Collier, "Top 5 Tips for Boosting GABA," Wellnicity.com (accessed May 12, 2020), https://www.wellnicity.com/articles/top-5-tips-for-boosting-gaba.

34. B. Lozoff et al., "Long-Lasting Neural and Behavioral Effects of Iron Deficiency in Infancy," *Nutrition Reviews*, vol. 64, no. 5, pt. 2 (May 2006): S34–43, doi: 10.1301/nr.2006.may.S34-S43.

35. H.R. Lieberman, "Amino Acid and Protein Requirements: Cognitive Performance, Stress, and Brain Function," in *The Role of Protein and Amino Acids in Sustaining and Enhancing Performance*, Institute of Medicine (Washington, D.C.: The National Academies Press, 1999), https://www.ncbi. nlm.nih.gov/books/NBK224629; A. Baranyi et al., "Branched-Chain Amino Acids as New Biomarkers of Major Depression: A Novel Neurobiology of Mood Disorder," *PLoS One*, vol. 11, no. 8 (2016), e0160542, doi: 10.1371/ journal.pone.0160542.

36. G. Wu, "Amino Acids: Metabolism, Functions, and Nutrition," *Amino Acids*, vol. 37, no. 1 (May 2009): 1–17, doi: 10.1007/s00726-009-0269-0.

37. P. Tessari, A. Lanti, and G. Mosca, "Essential Amino Acids: Master Regulators of Nutrition and Environmental Footprint?" *Scientific Reports*, vol. 6 (2016): 26074, doi: 10.1038/srep26074.

38. F. Mocci et al., "The Effect of Noise on Serum and Urinary Magnesium and Catecholamines in Humans," *Occupational Medicine*, vol. 51, no. 1 (February 2001): 56–61, doi: 10.1093/occmed/51.1.56.

39. B. Takase et al., "Effect of Chronic Stress and Sleep Deprivation on Both Flow-Mediated Dilation in the Brachial Artery and the Intracellular Magnesium Level in Humans," *Clinical Cardiology*, vol. 27, no. 4 (April 27, 2004): 223–7, doi: 10.1002/clc.4960270411.

40. G. Grases et al., "Anxiety and Stress Among Science Students: Study of Calcium and Magnesium Alterations," *Magnesium Research*, vol. 19, no. 2 (June 2006): 102–6, PMID: 16955721.

41. H.F. Chen and H.M. Su, "Exposure to a Maternal N-3 Fatty Acid-Deficient Diet During Brain Development Provokes Excessive Hypothalamic-Pituitary Adrenal Axis Responses to Stress and Behavioral Indices of Depression and Anxiety in Male Rat Offspring Later in Life," *Journal of Nutritional Biochemistry*, vol. 24, no. 1 (January 2013): 70–80, doi: 10.1016/j.jnutbio.2012.02.006.

42. J.J. Liu et al., "Omega-3 Polyunsaturated Fatty Acid (PUFA) Status in Major Depressive Disorder with Comorbid Anxiety Disorders," *Journal of Clinical Psychiatry*, vol. 74, no. 7 (July 2013): 732–8, doi: 10.4088/JCP.12m07970.

43. M.A. Pérez, G. Terreros, and A. Dagnino-Subiabre, "Long-Term Omega-3 Fatty Acid Supplementation Induces Anti-Stress Effects and Improves Learning in Rats," *Behavioral and Brain Functions*, vol. 9 (June 14, 2013): 25, doi: 10.1186/1744-9081-9-25; H.F. Chen and H.M. Su, "Fish Oil Supplementation of Maternal Rats on an N-3 Fatty Acid-Deficient Diet Prevents Depletion of Maternal Brain Regional Docosahexaenoic Acid Levels and Has a Postpartum Anxiolytic Effect," *Journal of Nutritional Biochemistry*, vol. 23, no. 3 (March 2013): 299–305, doi: 10.1016/j.jnutbio.2010.12.010; A. Wu et al., "Curcumin Boosts DHA in the Brain: Implications for the Prevention of Anxiety Disorders," *Biochimica et Biophysica Acta*, vol. 1852, no. 5 (May 2015): 951–61, doi: 10.1016/j.bbadis.2014.12.005.

44. A. Wu et al., "Curcumin Boosts DHA in the Brain: Implications for the Prevention of Anxiety Disorders," *Biochimica et Biophysica Acta*, vol. 1852, no. 5 (2015): 951–61, doi: 10.1016/j.bbadis.2014.12.005.

45. Y. Xu et al., "Novel Therapeutic Targets in Depression and Anxiety: Antioxidants as a Candidate Treatment," *Current Neuropharmacology*, vol. 12, no. 2 (March 2014): 108–119, doi: 10.2174/1570159X11666131120231448.

46. R. Krolow et al., "Oxidative Imbalance and Anxiety Disorders," *Current Neuropharmacology*, vol. 12, no. 2 (March 2014): 193–204, doi: 10.2174/1570159X11666131120223530.

47. M.H. Carlsen et al., "The Total Antioxidant Content of More than 3100 Foods, Beverages, Spices, Herbs and Supplements Used Worldwide," *Nutrition Journal*, vol. 9 (January 22, 2010): 3, doi: 10.1186/1475-2891-9-3.

48. Ibid.

49. A. Trichopoulou et al., "Vegetable and Fruit: The Evidence in Their Favour and the Public Health Perspective," *International Journal of Vitamin Nutritional Research*, vol. 73, no. 2 (March 2003): 63–9, doi: 10.1024/0300-9831.73.2.63.

50. J.R. Hibbeln et al., "Vegetarian Diets and Depressive Symptoms Among Men," *Journal of Affective Disorders*, vol. 225 (January 1, 2018): 13–17, doi: 10.1016/j.jad.2017.07.051.

51. M. Kornsteiner, I. Singer, and I. Elmadfa, "Very Low N-3 Long-chain Polyunsaturated Fatty Acid Status in Austrian Vegetarians and Vegans," *Annals of Nutrition and Metabolism*, vol. 52, no. 1 (2008): 37–47, doi: 10.1159/000118629.

52. A. Wu et al., "Curcumin Boosts DHA in the Brain: Implications for the Prevention of Anxiety Disorders," *Biochimica et Biophysica Acta,* vol. 1852, no. 5 (May 2015): 951–61, doi: 10.1016/j.bbadis.2014.12.005.

53. K.L. Brookie, G.I. Best, and T.S. Conner. "Intake of Raw Fruits and Vegetables Is Associated with Better Mental Health Than Intake of Processed Fruits and Vegetables," *Frontiers in Psychology,* vol. 9 (2018): 487, doi: 10.3389/fpsyg.2018.00487.

54. Ibid.

55. S. Salim, G. Chugh, and M. Asghar, "Inflammation in Anxiety," *Advances in Protein Chemistry and Structural Biology,* vol. 88 (2012): 1–25, doi: 10.1016/B978-0-12-398314-5.00001-5.

56. B.B. Aggarwhal and K.B. Harikumar, "Potential Therapeutic Effects of Curcumin, the Anti-Inflammatory Agent, Against Neurodegenerative, Cardiovascular, Pulmonary, Metabolic, Autoimmune and Neoplastic Diseases," *International Journal of Biochemistry & Cell Biology,* vol. 41, no. 1 (January 2009): 40–59, doi: 10.1016/j.biocel.2008.06.010.

57. G.M. Cole, B. Teter, and S.A. Frautschy, "Neuroprotective Effects of Curcumin," *Advances in Experimental Medicine and Biology,* vol. 595 (2007): 197–212, doi: 10.1007/978-0-387-46401-5_8.

Chapter 2

1. M. Bruguglio et al., "Dietary Neurotransmitters: A Narrative Review on Current Knowledge," *Nutrients,* vol. 10, no. 5 (May 2018): 591, doi: 10.3390/nu10050591.

2. Ibid.

3. E. Wang and M. Wink, "Chlorophyll Enhances Oxidative Stress Tolerance in *Caenorhabditis elegans* and Extends Its Lifespan," *PeerJ,* vol. 4 (April 7, 2016): e1879, doi: 10.7717/peerj.1879.

4. K.L. Brookie, G.I. Best, and T.S. Conner, "Intake of Raw Fruits and Vegetables Is Associated with Better Mental Health Than Intake of Processed Fruits and Vegetables," *Frontiers in Psychology,* vol. 9 (April 10, 2018), doi: 10.3389/fpsyg.2018.00487.

5. D.E. King et al., "Dietary Magnesium and C-Reactive Protein Levels," *Journal of the American College of Nutrition,* vol. 24, no. 5 (June 2005): 166–71, doi: 10.1080/07315724.2005.10719461; E.S. Ford and A.H. Mokdad, "Dietary Magnesium Intake in a National Sample of U.S. Adults," *Journal of Nutrition,* vol. 133, no. 9 (September 2003): 2879–82, doi: 10.1093/jn/133.9.2879; J.H. Dolega-Cieszkowski, J.P. Bobyn, and S.J. Whiting. "Dietary Intakes of Canadians in the 1990s Using Population-Weighted Data Derived from the Provincial Nutrition Surveys," *Applied Physiology, Nutrition, and Metabolism,* vol. 31, no. 6 (December 2006): 753–8, doi: 10.1139/h06-096.

6. P. Galan et al., "Dietary Magnesium Intake in a French Adult Population," *Magnesium Research*, vol. 10, no. 4 (December 1997): 321–8, PMID: 9513928.

7. N.B. Boyle, C. Lawton, and L. Dye, "The Effects of Magnesium Supplementation on Subjective Anxiety and Stress: A Systematic Review," Nutrients, vol. 9, no. 5 (May 2017), doi: 10.3390/nu9050429; M.L. Derom et al., "Magnesium and Depression: A Systematic Review," *Nutritional Neuroscience*, vol. 16, no. 5 (September 2013): 191–206, doi: 10.1179/1476830512Y.0000000044; G.A. Eby III and K.L. Eby, "Magnesium for Treatment-Resistant Depression: A Review and Hypothesis," *Medical Hypotheses*, vol. 74, no. 4 (April 2010): 649–60, doi: 10.1016/j.mehy.2009.10.051.

8. M.C. Morris et al., "Nutrients and Bioactives in Green Leafy Vegetables and Cognitive Decline: Prospective Study," *Neurology*, vol. 90, no. 3 (January 16, 2018): e214–22, doi: 10.1212/WNL.0000000000004815.

9. M.C. Morris et al., "Associations of Vegetable and Fruit Consumption with Age-Related Cognitive Change," *Neurology*, vol. 67 (October 24, 2006): 1370–76, doi: 10.1212/01.wnl.0000240224.38978.d8.

10. J.H. Kang, A. Ascherio, and F. Grodstein, "Fruit and Vegetable Consumption and Cognitive Decline in Aging Women," *Annals of Neurology*, vol. 57 (2005): 713–20, doi: 10.1002/ana.20476.

11. M.H. Carlsen et al., "The Total Antioxidant Content of More than 3100 Foods, Beverages, Spices, Herbs and Supplements Used Worldwide," *Nutrition Journal*, vol. 9 (2010): 3, doi: 10.1186/1475-2891-9-3.

12. P. Pribis, "Effects of Walnut Consumption on Mood in Young Adults: A Randomized Controlled Trial," *Nutrients*, vol. 8, no. 11 (November 2016): 668, doi: 10.3390/nu8110668.

13. L. Arab, R. Guo, and D. Elashoff, "Lower Depression Scores among Walnut Consumers in NHANES," *Nutrients*, vol. 11, no. 2 (February 2019): 275, doi: 10.3390/nu11020275.

14. A. Chauhan and V. Chauhan, "Beneficial Effects of Walnuts on Cognition and Brain Health," *Nutrients*, vol. 12, no. 2 (February 2020): 550, doi: 10.3390/nu12020550.

15. A. Wu et al., "Curcumin Boosts DHA in the Brain: Implications for the Prevention of Anxiety Disorders," *Biochimica et Biophysica Acta*, vol. 1852, no. 5 (May 2015): 251–61, doi: 10.1016/j.bbadis.2014.12.005.

16. S.K. Kulkarni and A. Dhir, "An Overview of Curcumin in Neurological Disorders," *Indian Journal of Pharmaceutical Sciences*, vol. 72, no. 2 (March–April 2010): 149–54, doi: 10.4103/0250-474X.65012.

17. B. Lee and H. Lee, "Systemic Administration of Curcumin Affect Anxiety-Related Behaviors in a Rat Model of Posttraumatic Stress Disorder via Activation of Serotonergic Systems," *Evidence-Based Complementary and Alternative Medicine*, vol. 2018 (June 19, 2018), 9041309, doi: 10.1155/2018/9041309.

18. N. Belhaj et al., "Anxiolytic-Like Effect of a Salmon Phospholipopeptidic Complex Composed of Polyunsaturated Fatty Acids and Bioactive Peptides," *Marine Drugs*, vol. 11, no. 11 (November 2013): 4294–4317, doi: 10.3390/md11114294.

19. A.L. Hansen et al., "Reduced Anxiety in Forensic Inpatients after a Long-Term Intervention with Atlantic Salmon," *Nutrients*, vol. 6, no. 12 (November 26, 2014): 5405–18, doi: 10.3390/nu6125405.

20. K. Ameer, "Avocado as a Major Dietary Source of Antioxidants and Its Preventive Role in Neurodegenerative Diseases," *Advances in Neurobiology*, vol. 12 (2016): 337–54, doi: 10.1007/978-3-319-28383-8_18.

21. A.P. de Oliveira et al., "Effect of Semisolid Formulation of *Persea americana* Mill (Avocado) Oil on Wound Healing in Rats," *Evidence-Based Complementary and Alternative Medicine*, vol. 2013 (March 2013): 472382, doi: 10.1155/2013/472382.

22. D.J. Bhuyan et al., "The Odyssey of Bioactive Compounds in Avocado (*Persea americana*) and Their Health Benefits," *Antioxidants*, vol. 8, no. 10 (October 2019): 426, doi: 10.3390/antiox8100426.

23. M.T. Murray and J. Pizzorno, *The Encyclopedia of Healing Foods* (New York: Simon and Schuster, 2010): 72.

24. J.J. Olivero Sr., "Cardiac Consequences of Electrolyte Imbalance," *Methodist DeBakey Cardiovascular Journal*, vol. 12, no. 2 (April–June 2016): 125–6, doi: 10.14797/mdcj-12-2-125.

25. D.J. Bhuyan et al., "The Odyssey of Bioactive Compounds in Avocado (*Persea americana*) and Their Health Benefits," *Antioxidants*, vol. 8, no. 10 (October 2019), doi: 10.3390/antiox8100426.

26. E. Coni et al., "Protective Effect of Oleuropein, an Olive Oil Biophenol, on Low Density Lipoprotein Oxidizability in Rabbits," *Lipids*, vol. 35, no. 1 (January 2000): 45–54, doi: 10.1007/s11745-000-0493-2.

27. B. Lee et al., "Oleuropein Reduces Anxiety-Like Responses by Activating of Serotonergic and Neuropeptide Y (NPY)-ergic Systems in a Rat model of Post-Traumatic Stress Disorder," *Animal Cells and Systems*, vol. 22, no. 2 (2018): 109–17, doi: 10.1080/19768354.2018.1426699.

28. T. Perveen et al., "Role of Monoaminergic System in the Etiology of Olive Oil Induced Antidepressant and Anxiolytic Effects in Rats," *ISRN Pharmacology*, vol. 2013 (2013): 615685, doi: 10.1155/2013/615685.

29. A.C. Logan, "Neurobehavioral Aspects of Omega-3 Fatty Acids: Possible Mechanisms and Therapeutic Value in Major Depression," *Alternative Medicine Review*, vol. 8, no. 4 (November 2003): 410–25, PMID: 14653768.

30. J. Bradbury, S.P. Myers, and C. Oliver, "An Adaptogenic Role for Omega-3 Fatty Acids in Stress: A Randomised Placebo-Controlled Double-Blind Intervention Study (Pilot) [ISRCTN22569553]," *Nutrition Journal*, vol. 3 (November 2004): 20, doi: 10.1186/1475-2891-3-20.

31. F. Paiva-Martins and M.H. Gordon, "Interactions of Ferric Ions with Olive Oil Phenolic Compounds," *Journal of Agriculture and Food Chemistry*, vol. 53, no. 7 (April 6, 2005): 2704–9, doi: 10.1021/jf0481094.

32. F. Hadrich et al., "Evaluation of Hypocholesterolemic Effect of Oleuropein in Cholesterol-Fed Rats," *Chemico-Biological Interactions*, vol. 252 (May 25, 2016): 54–60, doi: 10.1016/j.cbi.2016.03.026.

33. K. Zeratsky, "I've heard the term 'functional foods,' but I don't know what it means. Can you explain?" Mayo Clinic *Healthy Lifestyle* blog (accessed May 10, 2020), https://www.mayoclinic.org/healthy-lifestyle/nutrition -and-healthy-eating/expert-answers/functional-foods/faq-20057816.

34. S.K. Yeap, "Antistress and Antioxidant Effects of Virgin Coconut Oil in Vivo," *Experimental and Therapeutic Medicine*, vol. 9, no. 1 (January 2015): 39–42, doi: 10.3892/etm.2014.2045.

35. J.L. Platero et al., "The Impact of Coconut Oil and Epigallocatechin Gallate on the Levels of IL-6, Anxiety and Disability in Multiple Sclerosis Patients," *Nutrients*, vol. 12, no. 2 (January 23, 2020): 305, doi: 10.3390/nu12020305.

36. D.C. da Silva et al., "Can Coconut Oil and Treadmill Exercise During the Critical Period of Brain Development Ameliorate Stress-Related Effects on Anxiety-Like Behavior and Episodic-Like Memory in Young Rats?" *Food & Function*, vol. 9, no. 3 (March 1, 2018): 1492–9, doi: 10.1039/c7fo01516j.

37. J.W. Fahey, Y. Zhang, and P. Talalay, "Broccoli Sprouts: An Exceptionally Rich Source of Inducers of Enzymes that Protect Against Chemical Carcinogens," *Proceedings of the National Academy of Sciences (PNAS)*, vol. 94, no. 19 (September 16, 1997): 10367–72, doi: 10.1073/pnas.94.19.10367.

38. Y. Yaqishita et al., "Broccoli or Sulforaphane: Is It the Source or Dose That Matters?" *Molecules*, vol. 24, no. 19 (October 6, 2019): 3593, doi: 10.3390/ molecules24193593.

39. D.A. Moreno et al., "Chemical and Biological Characterisation of Nutraceutical Compounds of Broccoli," *Journal of Pharmaceutical and Biomedical Analysis*, vol. 41, no. 5 (August 28, 2006): 1508–22, doi: 10.1016/j. jpba.2006.04.003.

40. G.S. Stoewsand, "Bioactive Organosulfur Phytochemicals in *Brassica oleracea* Vegetables: A Review," *Food and Chemical Toxicology*, vol. 33, no. 6 (June 1995): 537–43, doi: 10.1016/0278-6915(95)00017-v.

41. M. Valko et al., "Free Radicals and Antioxidants in Normal Physiological Functions and Human Disease," *International Journal of Biochemical Cell Biology*, vol. 39, no. 1 (2007): 44–84, PMID: 23675073; J.H. Hwang and S.B. Lim, "Antioxidant and Anti-Inflammatory Activities of Broccoli Florets in LPS-Stimulated RAW 264.7 Cells," *Preventive Nutrition and Food Science*, vol. 19, no. 2 (June 2014): 89–97, doi: 10.3746/pnf.2014.19.2.089.

42. M.M. Kushad et al., "Variation of Glucosinolates in Vegetable Crops of *Brassica oleracea*," *Journal of Agriculture and Food Chemistry*, vol. 47, no. 4 (April 1999): 1541–8, doi: 10.1021/jf980985s.

43. A. Yanaka, "Daily Intake of Broccoli Sprouts Normalizes Bowel Habits in Human Healthy Subjects," *Journal of Clinical Biochemistry and Nutrition*, vol. 62, no. 1 (January 2018): 75–82, doi: 10.3164/jcbn.17-42.

44. T. La Forge, "7 Everyday Tonics that Help Your Body Adjust to Stress and Anxiety," *Healthline* (accessed April 22, 2020), https://www.healthline.com /health/food-nutrition/drinks-for-stress-anxiety#maca.

45. A.M. Bode and Z. Dong, "The Amazing and Mighty Ginger," chap. 7 in *Herbal Medicine: Biomolecular and Clinical Aspects, 2nd ed.*, eds. I.F.F. Benzie and S. Wachtel-Galor (Boca Raton, FL: CRC Press/Taylor & Francis, 2011), PMID: 22593941.

46. S.L. Vishwakarma et al., "Anxiolytic and Antiemetic Activity of *Zingiber officinale*," *Phytotherapy Research*, vol. 16, no. 7 (November 2002): 621–6, doi: 10.1002/ptr.948; F. Fatemeh, M. Modaresi, and I. Sajjadian, "The Effects of Ginger Extract and Diazepam on Anxiety Reduction in Animal Model," *Indian Journal of Pharmaceutical Education and Research*, vol. 51, no. 3 (July– September 2017): s159–62, doi: 10.5530/ijper.51.3s.4.

47. G.N. Martin, "Human Electroencephalographic (EEG) Response to Olfactory Stimulation: Two Experiments Using the Aroma of Food," *International Journal of Psychophysiology*, vol. 30, no. 3 (November 1998): 287–302, doi: 10.1016/s0167-8760(98)00025-7.

48. A.A. Sunni and R. Latif, "Effects of Chocolate Intake on Perceived Stress: A Controlled Clinical Study," *International Journal of Health Sciences*, vol. 8, no. 4 (October 2014): 393–401, PMID: 25780358.

49. F.P. Martin et al., "Everyday Eating Experiences of Chocolate and Non-Chocolate Snacks Impact Postprandial Anxiety, Energy and Emotional States," *Nutrients*, vol. 4, no. 6 (June 2012): 554–67, doi: 10.3390/nu4060554.

50. A.A. Sunni and R. Latif, "Effects of Chocolate Intake on Perceived Stress: A Controlled Clinical Study," *International Journal of Health Sciences*, vol. 8, no. 4 (October 2014): 393–401, PMID: 25780358.

51. Ibid.

52. A. Nehlig, "The Neuroprotective Effects of Cocoa Flavanol and Its Influence on Cognitive Performance," *British Journal of Clinical Pharmacology*, vol. 75, no. 3 (March 2013): 716–27, doi: 10.1111/j.1365-2125.2012.04378.x.

53. F.P. Martin et al., "Metabolic Effects of Dark Chocolate Consumption on Energy, Gut Microbiota, and Stress-Related Metabolism in Free-Living Subjects," *Journal of Proteome Research*, vol. 8, no. 12 (December 2009): 5568–79, doi: 10.1021/pr900607v.

54. A.B. Scholey et al., "Consumption of Cocoa Flavanols Results in Acute Improvements in Mood and Cognitive Performance During Sustained Mental Effort," *Journal of Psychopharmacology*, vol. 24, no. 10 (October 2010): 1505–14, doi: 10.1177/0269881109106923.

55. B.A. Golomb, S. Koperski, and H.L. White, "Association Between More Frequent Chocolate Consumption and Lower Body Mass Index," *Archives of Internal Medicine*, vol. 172, no. 6 (March 26, 2012): 519–21, doi: 10.1001/archinternmed.2011.2100.

56. P. Bhatia and N. Singh, "Homocysteine Excess: Delineating the Possible Mechanism of Neurotoxicity and Depression," *Fundamental & Clinical Pharmacology*, vol. 29, no. 6 (December 2015): 522–8, doi: 10.1111/fcp.12145; M.O. Ebesunun et al., "Elevated Plasma Homocysteine in Association with Decreased Vitamin B(12), Folate, Serotonin, Lipids and Lipoproteins in Depressed Patients," *African Journal of Psychiatry*, vol. 15, no. 1 (January 2012): 25–9, doi: 10.4314/ajpsy.v15i1.3.

57. M.H. Carlsen et al., "The Total Antioxidant Content of More than 3100 Foods, Beverages, Spices, Herbs and Supplements Used Worldwide," *Nutrition Journal*, vol. 9 (2010): 3, doi: 10.1186/1475-2891-9-3.

58. Ibid.

59. R.H.X. Wong et al., "Chronic Effects of a Wild Green Oat Extract Supplementation on Cognitive Performance in Older Adults: A Randomised, Double-Blind, Placebo-Controlled, Crossover Trial," *Nutrients*, vol. 4, no. 5 (May 2012): 331–42, doi: 10.3390/nu4050331; K. Abascal and E. Yarnell, "Nervine Herbs for Treating Anxiety," *Alternative and Complementary Therapies*, vol. 10, no. 6 (December 14, 2004): 309–15, doi: 10.1089/act.2004.10.309; W. Guo et al., "Avenanthramides, Polyphenols from Oats, Inhibit IL-1beta-induced NF-kappaB Activation in Endothelial Cells," *Free Radical Biology and Medicine*, vol. 44, no. 3 (February 1, 2008): 415–29, doi: 10.1016/j.freeradbiomed.2007.10.036.

60. W. Dimpfel, C. Storni, and M.J. Verbruggen, "Ingested Oat Herb (*Avena sativa*) Changes EEG Spectral Frequencies in Healthy Subjects," *Alternative and Complementary Medicine*, vol. 17, no. 5 (May 2011): 427–34, doi: 10.1089/acm.2010.0143.

61. W. Guo et al., "Avenanthramides, Polyphenols from Oats, Inhibit IL-1beta-induced NF-kappaB Activation in Endothelial Cells," *Free Radical Biology and Medicine*, vol. 44, no. 3 (February 1, 2008): 415–29, doi: 10.1016/j.freeradbiomed.2007.10.036.

Chapter 3

1. S.E. Lakhan and K.F. Vieira, "Nutritional and Herbal Supplements for Anxiety and Anxiety-Related Disorders: Systematic Review," *Nutrition Journal*, vol. 9 (October 7, 2010): 42, doi: 10.1186/1475-2891-9-42.

2. M. Stein, S.E. Keller, and S.J. Schleifer. "Immune System: Relationship to Anxiety Disorders," *Psychiatric Clinics of North America*, vol. 11, no. 2 (June 1988): 349–60, PMID: 3047704.

3. M.M. Dias et al., "Anti-Inflammatory Activity of Polyphenolics from Açai (*Euterpe oleracea* Martius) in Intestinal Myofibroblasts CCD-18Co Cells," *Food & Function*, vol. 6, no. 10 (October 2015): 3249–56, doi: 10.1039/c5fo00278h.

4. A.K. Marchado, "Neuroprotective Effects of Açaí (*Euterpe oleracea* Mart.) against Rotenone in Vitro Exposure," *Oxidative Medicine and Cellular Longevity* (2016): 8940850, doi: 10.1155/2016/8940850.

5. S.S. Dutta, "Hippocampus Functions," *News-Medical* (August 20, 2019), https://www.news-medical.net/health/Hippocampus-Functions.aspx.

6. M. Sriga et al., "Oral Treatment with L-Lysine and L-Arginine Reduces Anxiety and Basal Cortisol Levels in Healthy Humans," *Biomedical Research*, vol. 28, no. 2 (April 2007): 85–90, doi: 10.2220/biomedres.28.85.

7. G. Sandrini et al., "Effectiveness of Ibuprofen-Arginine in the Treatment of Acute Migraine Attacks," *International Journal of Clinical Pharmacology Research*, vol. 18, no. 3 (1998): 145–50, PMID: 9825271.

8. J.R. McKnight et al., "Beneficial Effects of L-Arginine on Reducing Obesity: Potential Mechanisms and Important Implications for Human Health," *Amino Acids*, vol. 39, no. 2 (2010): 349–57, doi: 10.1007/s00726-010-0598-z.

9. S. Srinongkote et al., "A Diet Fortified with L-Lysine and L-Arginine Reduces Plasma Cortisol and Blocks Anxiogenic Response to Transportation in Pigs," *Nutritional Neuroscience*, vol. 6, no. 5 (October 2003): 283–9, doi: 10.1080/10284150310001614661.

10. D. Christmas, S. Hood, and D. Nutt. "Potential Novel Anxiolytic Drugs," *Current Pharmaceutical Design*, vol. 14, no. 33 (2008): 3534–46, doi: 10.2174/138161208786848775.

11. "What Is Serotonin and What Does It Do?" *Medical News Today* (accessed April 29, 2020), https://www.medicalnewstoday.com/articles /232248#what-is-serotonin?

12. L.R. Juneja et al., "L-Theanine: A Unique Amino Acid of Green Tea and Its Relaxation Effect in Humans," *Trends in Food Science & Technology*, vol. 10, nos. 6–7 (1999): 199–204, doi: 10.1016/S0924-2244(99)00044-8.

13. A.C. Nobre, A. Rao, and G.N. Owen. "L-Theanine, a Natural Constituent in Tea, and Its Effect on Mental State," *Asia Pacific Journal of Clinical Nutrition*, vol. 17, supp. 1 (2008): 167–8, PMID: 18296328.

14. F.L. Sakamoto et al., "Psychotropic Effects of L-theanine and Its Clinical Properties: From the Management of Anxiety and Stress to a Potential Use in Schizophrenia," *Pharmacological Research*, vol. 147 (September 2019): 104395, doi: 10.1016/j.phrs.2019.104395.

15. T.S. Sathyanarayana Rao and V.K. Yeragani, "Hypertensive Crisis and Cheese," *Indian Journal of Psychiatry*, vol. 51, no. 1 (January–March 2009): 65–6, doi: 10.4103/0019-5545.44910.

16. "Compound Summary: Tyrosine," U.S. National Library of Medicine (accessed April 10, 2020), https://pubchem.ncbi.nlm.nih.gov/compound/L-tyrosine; J.D. Fernstrom and M.H. Fernstrom, "Tyrosine, Phenylalanine, and Catecholamine Synthesis and Function in the Brain," *Journal of Nutrition*, vol. 137, no. 6, supp. 1 (June 2007): 1539S–47S, doi: 10.1093/jn/137.6.1539S.

17. R. Mullur, Y.Y. Liu, and G.A. Brent, "Thyroid Hormone Regulation of Metabolism," *Physiological Reviews*, vol. 94, no. 2 (April 2014): 355–82, doi: 10.1152/physrev.00030.2013.

18. S.N. Young, "L-Tyrosine to Alleviate the Effects of Stress?" *Journal of Psychiatry & Neuroscience*, vol. 32, no. 3 (May 2007): 224, PMID: 17476368.

19. Report of a Joint WHO/FAO/UNU Expert Consultation, "Protein and Amino Acid Requirements in Human Beings," World Health Organization (2002), https://apps.who.int/iris/handle/10665/43411.

20. Gavin Van De Walle, "Tyrosine: Benefits, Side Effects and Dosage," *Healthline* (February 1, 2018), https://www.healthline.com/nutrition/tyrosine.

21. K. Chandrasekhar, J. Kapoor, and S. Anishetty. "A Prospective, Randomized Double-Blind, Placebo-Controlled Study of Safety and Efficacy of a High-Concentration Full-Spectrum Extract of Ashwagandha Root in Reducing Stress and Anxiety in Adults," *Indian Journal of Psychological Medicine*, vol. 34, no. 3 (July 2012): 255–62, doi: 10.4103/0253-7176.106022.

22. S.R. Fauce et al., "Telomerase-Based Pharmacologic Enhancement of Antiviral Function of Human CD8+ T Lymphocytes," *Journal of Immunology*, vol. 181, no. 10 (November 15, 2008): 7400–6, doi: 10.4049/jimmunol.181.10.7400.

23. B.R. Hoobler, "Symptomatology of Vitamin B Deficiency in Infants," *JAMA*, vol. 91, no. 5 (August 4, 1928): 307–10, doi: 10.1001/jama.1928 .02700050013005.

24. "Vitamin B12: Fact Sheet for Consumers," National Institutes of Health, Office of Dietary Supplements (accessed April 9, 2020), https://ods.od.nih .gov/factsheets/VitaminB12-Consumer.

25. L.M. Young et al., "A Systematic Review and Meta-Analysis of B Vitamin Supplementation on Depressive Symptoms, Anxiety, and Stress: Effects on Healthy and 'At-Risk' Individuals," *Nutrients*, vol. 11, no. 9 (September 16, 2019): 2232, doi: 10.3390/nu11092232.

26. D. Lonsdale and R.J. Shamberger, "Red Cell Transketolase as an Indicator of Nutritional Deficiency?" *American Journal of Clinical Nutrition*, vol. 33, no. 2 (February 1980): 205–11, doi: 10.1093/ajcn/33.2.205.

27. Fondriest Environmental, Inc., "Algae, Phytoplankton and Chlorophyll," Fundamentals of Environmental Measurements (October 22, 2014), https://www.fondriest.com/environmental-measurements/parameters/water-quality/algae-phytoplankton-chlorophyll.

28. "Blue-Green Algae," WebMD (accessed April 8, 2020), https://www.webmd.com/vitamins/ai/ingredientmono-923/blue-green-algae.

29. S.H. Lee et al., "Six-Week Supplementation with Chlorella Has Favorable Impact on Antioxidant Status in Korean Male Smokers," *Nutrition*, vol. 26, no. 2 (February 2010): 175–83, doi: 10.1016/j.nut.2009.03.010.

30. P.D. Karkos et al., "Spirulina in Clinical Practice: Evidence-Based Human Applications," *Evidence-Based Complementary and Alternative Medicine*, vol. 2011 (October 19, 2010): 531053, doi: 10.1093/ecam/nen058.

31. M. Watson, "The History of Spirulina: From Nutrition Provider to Vivid Color," Watson, Inc. blog (April 25, 2017), https://blog.watson-inc.com/nutri-knowledge/the-history-of-spirulina-from-nutrition-provider-to-vivid-color.

32. P.D. Karkos et al., "Spirulina in Clinical Practice: Evidence-Based Human Applications," *Evidence-Based Complementary and Alternative Medicine*, vol. 2011 (October 19, 2010): 531053, doi: 10.1093/ecam/nen058.

33. S. Lordan, R.P. Ross, and C. Stanton, "Marine Bioactives as Functional Food Ingredients: Potential to Reduce the Incidence of Chronic Diseases," *Marine Drugs*, vol. 9, no. 6 (2011): 1056–1100, doi: 10.3390/md9061056.

34. X. Tian et al., "Neuroprotective effects of *Arctium lappa* L. Roots Against Glutamate-Induced Oxidative Stress by Inhibiting Phosphorylation of p38, JNK and ERK 1/2 MAPKs in PC12 Cells," *Environmental Toxicology and Pharmacology*, vol. 38, no. 1 (July 2014): 189–98, doi: 10.1016/j.etap.2014.05.017.

35. S. Shannon et al., "Cannabidiol in Anxiety and Sleep: A Large Case Series," *Permanente Journal*, vol. 23 (January 7, 2019): 18–41, doi: 10.7812/TPP/18-041.

36. Alan Carter, "Does CBD Show Up on a Drug Test?" *Healthline* (April 24, 2019), https://www.healthline.com/health/does-cbd-show-up-on-a-drug-test.

37. E. M. Blessing et al., "Cannabidiol as a Potential Treatment for Anxiety Disorders," *Neurotherapeutics*, vol. 12, no. 4 (September 4, 2015): 825–36, doi: 10.1007/s13311-015-0387-1.

38. S.A. Stoner, "Effects of Marijuana on Mental Health: Anxiety Disorders," Alcohol & Drug Abuse Institute, University of Washington, June 2017, http://adai.uw.edu/pubs/pdf/2017mjanxiety.pdf.

39. W. Hall and N. Solowij, "Adverse Effects of Cannabis," *Lancet*, vol. 352, no. 9140 (November 14, 1998): 1611–6, doi: 10.1016/S0140-6736(98)05021-1.

40. M. Underner et al., "Cannabis Smoking and Lung Cancer" [article in French], *Revue des Maladies Respiratoires*, vol. 31, no. 6 (June 2014): 488–98, doi: 10.1016/j.rmr.2013.12.002.

41. J.J. Mao et al., "Long-Term Chamomile Therapy of Generalized Anxiety Disorder: A Study Protocol for a Randomized, Double-Blind, Placebo-Controlled Trial," *Journal of Clinical Trials*, vol. 4, no. 5 (November 2014): 188, doi: 10.4172/2167-0870.1000188.

42. E. Wang and M. Wink. "Chlorophyll Enhances Oxidative Stress Tolerance in *Caenorhabditis elegans* and Extends Its Lifespan," *PeerJ*, vol. 4 (April 7, 2016): e1879, doi: 10.7717/peerj.1879.

43. M. Nakamura et al., "Low Zinc, Copper, and Manganese Intake is Associated with Depression and Anxiety Symptoms in the Japanese Working Population: Findings from the Eating Habit and Well-Being Study," *Nutrients*, vol. 11, no. 4 (April 15, 2019): e847, doi: 10.3390/nu11040847.

44. L.A. Dykman and N.G. Khlebtsov, "Gold Nanoparticles in Biology and Medicine: Recent Advances and Prospects," *Acta Naturae*, vol. 3, no. 2 (April–June 2011): 34–55, PMID: 22649683.

45. B.S. Zolnik et al., "Nanoparticles and the Immune System," *Endocrinology*, vol. 151, no. 2 (February 2010): 458–65, doi: 10.1210/en.2009-1082.

46. A. Van Arsdall and T. Graham, eds., *Herbs and Healers from the Ancient Mediterranean through the Medieval West: Essays in Honor of John M. Riddle* (New York: Routledge, 2016): 290.

47. K. Hu et al., "Neuroprotective Effect of Gold Nanoparticles Composites in Parkinson's Disease Model," *Nanomedicine: Nanotechnology, Biology and Medicine*, vol. 14, no. 4 (June 2018): 1123–36, doi: 10.1016/j.nano.2018.01.020.

48. R. Mukherjee, P.K. Dash, and G.C. Ram, "Immunotherapeutic Potential of *Ocimum sanctum* (L) in Bovine Subclinical Mastitis," *Research in Veterinary Science*, vol. 79, no. 1 (2005): 37–43, doi: 10.1016/j.rvsc.2004.11.001.

49. S. Sampath et al., "Holy Basil (*Ocimum sanctum* Linn.) Leaf Extract Enhances Specific Cognitive Parameters in Healthy Adult Volunteers: A Placebo Controlled Study," *Indian Journal of Physiology and Pharmacology*, vol. 59, no. 1 (January–March 2015): 69–77, PMID: 26571987.

50. N. Jamshidi and M.M. Cohen, "The Clinical Efficacy and Safety of Tulsi in Humans: A Systematic Review of the Literature," *Evidence-Based Complementary and Alternative Medicine*, vol. 1 (March 16, 2017): 1–13, doi: 10.1155/2017/9217567.

51. R.C. Saxena et al., "Efficacy of an Extract of *Ocimum tenuiflorum* (OciBest) in the Management of General Stress: A Double-Blind, Placebo-Controlled Study," *Evidence-Based Complementary and Alternative Medicine* (October 3, 2011), 894509, doi: 10.1155/2012/894509.

52. J. Cawte, "Psychoactive Substances of the South Seas: Betel, Kava, and Pituri," *Australian and New Zealand Journal of Psychiatry*, vol. 19, no. 1 (March 1995): 83–7, doi: 10.3109/00048678509158818.

53. N.R. Bruner and K.G. Anderson, "Discriminative-Stimulus and Time-Course Effects of Kava-Kava (*Piper methysticum*) in Rats," *Pharmacology, Biochemistry, and Behavior*, vol. 92, no. 2 (April 2009): 297–303, doi: 10.1016/j.pbb.2008.12.017.

54. H.P. Volz and M. Kieser, "Kava-Kava Extract WS 1490 versus Placebo in Anxiety Disorders—A Randomized Placebo-Controlled 25-week Outpatient Trial," *Pharmacopsychiatry*, vol. 30, no. 1 (1997): 1–5, doi: 10.1055/s-2007-979474.

55. A. Scholey et al., "Anti-Stress Effects of Lemon Balm-Containing Foods," *Nutrients*, vol. 6, no. 11 (November 2014): 4805–21, doi: 10.3390/nu6114805.

56. C. Bhatt et al., "Synergistic Potentiation of Anti-Anxiety Activity of Valerian and Alprazolam by Liquorice," *Indian Journal of Pharmacology*, vol. 45, no. 2 (March–April 2013): 202–3, doi: 10.4103/0253-7613.108328.

57. M.J. Cho et al., "Comparison of the Effect of Three Licorice Varieties on Cognitive Improvement *via* an Amelioration of Neuroinflammation in Lipopolysaccharide-Induced Mice," *Nutrition Research and Practice*, vol. 12, no. 3 (June 2018):191–8, doi: 10.4162/nrp.2018.12.3.191.

58. N.B. Boyle, C. Lawton, and L. Dye, "The Effects of Magnesium Supplementation on Subjective Anxiety and Stress: A Systematic Review," *Nutrients*, vol. 9, no. 5 (May 2017): 429, doi: 10.3390/nu9050429.

59. M.P. Guerrera, S.L. Volpe, and J.J. Mao, "Therapeutic Uses of Magnesium," *American Family Physician*, vol. 80, no. 2 (July 15, 2009): 157–62, PMID: 19621856.

60. S.B. Sartori et al., "Magnesium Deficiency Induces Anxiety and HPA Axis Dysregulation: Modulation by Therapeutic Drug Treatment," *Neuropharmacology*, vol. 62, no. 1 (January 2012): 304–12, doi: 10.1016/j.neuropharm.2011.07.027.

61. S. Cornish and L. Mehl-Medrona, "The Role of Vitamins and Minerals in Psychiatry," *Integrative Medicine Insights*, vol. 3 (2008): 33–42, PMID: 21614157.

62. E.K. Tarleton et al., "Role of Magnesium Supplementation in the Treatment of Depression: A Randomized Clinical Trial," *PLoS One*, vol. 12, no. 6 (June 27, 2017): e0180067, doi: 10.1371/journal.pone.0180067.

63. D.X. Tan et al., "Melatonin: A Potent, Endogenous Hydroxyl Radical Scavenger," *Endocrine Journal*, vol. 1 (1993): 57–60.

64. "Melatonin and Sleep," National Sleep Foundation (accessed April 29, 2020), https://www.sleepfoundation.org/articles/melatonin-and-sleep.

65. M.V. Hansen et al., "Melatonin for Pre- and Postoperative Anxiety in Adults," *Cochrane Database of Systematic Reviews*, vol. 4 (April 2015): CD009861, doi: 10.1002/14651858.CD009861.pub2.

66. Catherine Saint Louis, "Dessert, Laid-Back and Legal," *New York Times* (May 14, 2011O, https://www.nytimes.com/2011/05/15/us/15lazycakes.html.

67. Sree Roy, "Despite FDA Warning Letters, Melatonin-laced Food and Beverage Market Grows," Sleep Review (Aug 25, 2014), https://www.sleepreviewmag .com/sleep-disorders/insomnia/despite-fda-warning-letters-melatonin-laced -food-beverage-market-grows.

68. "As Melatonin Use Rises, So Do Safety Concerns," WebMD (November 12, 2018), https://www.webmd.com/sleep-disorders/news/20181112 /as-melatonin-use-rises-so-do-safety-concerns.

69. G. Grosso et al., "Omega-3 Fatty Acids and Depression: Scientific Evidence and Biological Mechanisms," *Oxidative Medicine and Cellular Longevity*, vol. 2014 (2014): 313570, doi: 10.1155/2014/313570.

70. K. Dhawan et al., "Correct Identification of *Passiflora incarnata* Linn., a Promising Herbal Anxiolytic and Sedative," *Journal of Medicinal Food*, vol. 4, no. 3 (Autumn 2001): 137–44, doi: 10.1089/109662001753165710.

71. K. Dhawan, S. Kumar, and A. Sharma, "Antianxiety Studies on Extracts of *Passiflora incarnata* Linneaus," *Journal of Ethnopharmacology*, vol. 78, nos. 2–3 (December 2001): 165–70, doi: 10.1016/s0378-8741(01)00339-7.

72. S. Akhondzadeh et al., "Passionflower in the Treatment of Generalized Anxiety: A Pilot Double-Blind Randomized Controlled Trial with Oxazepam," *Journal of Clinical Pharmacy and Therapeutics*, vol. 26, no. 5 (October 2001): 363–7, doi: 10.1046/j.1365-2710.2001.00367.x; M. Bourin et al., "A Combination of Plant Extracts in the Treatment of Outpatients with Adjustment Disorder with Anxious Mood: Controlled Study versus Placebo," *Fundamental & Clinical Pharmacology*, vol. 11, no. 2 (August 26, 2009): 127–32, doi: 10.1111/j.1472-8206.1997.tb00179.x.

73. S. Akhondzadeh et al., "Passionflower in the Treatment of Generalized Anxiety: A Pilot Double-Blind Randomized Controlled Trial with Oxazepam," *Journal of Clinical Pharmacy and Therapeutics*, vol. 26, no. 5 (October 2001): 363–7, doi: 10.1046/j.1365-2710.2001.00367.x.

74. American Gastroenterological Association, "AGA's Interpretation of the Latest Probiotics Research" (September 26, 2018), https://gastro.org/press -releases/agas-interpretation-of-the-latest-probiotics-research; "Should You Take Probiotics?" *Harvard Health Letter* (April 2015, updated August 20, 2019), https://www.health.harvard.edu/staying-healthy/should-you-take -probiotics.

75. "Rhodiola," National Center for Integrative and Complementary Health (accessed April 10, 2020), https://www.nccih.nih.gov/health/rhodiola.

76. M. Cropley, A.P. Banks, and J. Boyle, "The Effects of *Rhodiola rosea* L. Extract on Anxiety, Stress, Cognition, and Other Mood Symptoms," *Phytotherapy Research*, vol. 29, no. 12 (December 2015): 1934–9, doi: 10.1002/ptr.5486.

77. "Schisandra," RxList (September 17, 2019), https://www.rxlist.com /schisandra/supplements.htm.

78. W.W. Chen et al., "Pharmacological Studies on the Anxiolytic Effect of Standardized Schisandra Lignans Extract on Restraint-Stressed Mice," *Phytomedicine*, vol. 18, no. 13 (October 15, 2011): 1144–7, doi: 10.1016/j. phymed.2011.06.004.

79. K. Linde et al., "St John's Wort for Depression: An Overview and Meta-Analysis of Randomised Clinical Trials," *BMJ*, vol. 13, no. 7052 (August 3, 1996): 253–8, doi: 10.1136/bmj.313.7052.253.

80. "St. John's Wort," Mayo Clinic (Ocober 13, 2017), https://www.mayoclinic .org/drugs-supplements-st-johns-wort/art-20362212.

81. H.P. Volz et al., "St John's Wort Extract (LI 160) in Somatoform Disorders: Results of a Placebo-Controlled Trial," *Psychopharmacology*, vol. 164 (November 2002): 294–300, doi: 10.1007/s00213-002-1171-6.

82. "St. John's Wort and Depression: In Depth," National Center for Complementary and Integrative Health (NCCIH) (December 2017), https:// www.nccih.nih.gov/health/st-johns-wort-and-depression-in-depth.

83. "Colloid," Wikipedia.com (accessed April 10, 2020), https://en.wikipedia.org /wiki/Colloid.

84. Edward Group, "5 Things You Must Know about Colloidal Silver," Global Healing Center (October 5, 2015), https://www.globalhealingcenter .com/natural-health/5-things-must-know-colloidal-silver.

85. R.S. Bell and T.M. Bollinger, *Unlock the Power to Heal* (City, UT: Infinity 510 Squared Partners, 2014): 87.

86. K. Morrill et al., "Spectrum of Antimicrobial Activity Associated with Ionic Colloidal Silver," *Journal of Alternative and Complementary Medicine*, vol. 19, no. 3 (March 2013): 224–31, doi: 10.1089/acm.2011.0681.

87. A.J. Russo, "Decreased Zinc and Increased Copper in Individuals with Anxiety," *Nutrition and Metabolic Insights*, vol. 4 (February 7, 2011): 1–5, doi: 10.4137/NMI.S6349.

Chapter 4

1. J. Bouayoud, H. Rammal, and R. Soulimani. "Oxidative Stress and Anxiety," *Oxidative Medicine and Cellular Longevity*, vol. 2, no. 2 (April–June 2009): 63–7, doi: 10.4161/oxim.2.2.7944.

2. S. Robertson, "What is Neurotoxicity?" News Medical Life Sciences (September 16, 2017), https://www.news-medical.net/health/What-is -Neurotoxicity.aspx.

3. L.C. Dolan, R.A. Matulka, and G.A. Burdock, "Naturally Occurring Food Toxins," *Toxins*, vol. 2, no. 9 (September 2010): 2289–332, doi: 10.3390/ toxins2092289.

4. M.R. Hilimire, J.E. DeVylder, and C.A. Forestell, "Fermented Foods, Neuroticism, and Social Anxiety: An Interaction Model," *Psychiatry Research*, vol. 28, no. 2 (August 15, 2015): 203–8, doi: 10.1016/j.psychres.2015.04.023.

5. C.J.K. Wallace and R. Miley, "The Effects of Probiotics on Depressive Symptoms in Humans: A Systematic Review," *Annals of General Psychiatry*, vol. 16 (2017): 14, doi: 10.1186/s12991-017-0138-2.

6. A. Gea et al., "Alcohol Intake, Wine Consumption and the Development of Depression: The PREDIMED Study," *BMC Medicine*, vol. 11 (August 20, 2013): 192, doi: 10.1186/1741-7015-11-192.

7. C. Baum-Baicker, "The Psychological Benefits of Moderate Alcohol Consumption: A Review of the Literature," *Drug and Alcohol Dependence*, vol. 15, no. 4 (August 1985): 305–22, doi: 10.1016/0376-8716(85)90008-0.

8. G.-Esquinas et al., "Moderate Alcohol Drinking Is Not Associated with Risk of Depression in Older Adults," *Scientific Reports*, vol. 8 (2018): 11512, doi: 10.1038/s41598-018-29985-4.

9. M. Dow, "How to Beat Midlife Brain Fog," DrMikeDow.com (accessed May 1, 2020), https://drmikedow.com/how-to-beat-midlife-brain-fog.

10. J. Kim and K.W. Lee, "Coffee and Its Active Compounds are Neuroprotective," chap. 46 in *Coffee in Health and Disease Prevention*, V.R. Preedy, ed. (Cambridge, MA: Academic Press, 2015), doi: 10.1016/ B978-0-12-409517-5.00046-2.

11. M.A. Lee, O.G. Cameron, and J.F. Greden, "Anxiety and Caffeine Consumption in People with Anxiety Disorders," *Psychiatry Research*, vol. 15, no. 3 (July 1985): 211–7, doi: 10.1016/0165-1781(85)90078-2.

12. J.L. Temple et al., "The Safety of Ingested Caffeine: A Comprehensive Review," *Frontiers in Psychology*, vol. 8 (May 26, 2017): 80, doi: 10.3389/ fpsyt.2017.00080.

13. G. Richards and A. Smith, "Caffeine Consumption and Self-assessed Stress, Anxiety, and Depression in Secondary School Children," *Journal of Psychopharmacology*, vol. 29, no. 12 (December 2015): 1236–47, doi: 10.1177/0269881115612404.

14. F. Visioli and A. Strata, "Milk, Dairy Products, and Their Functional Effects in Humans: A Narrative Review of Recent Evidence," *Advances in Nutrition*, vol. 5, no. 2 (March 2014): 131–43, doi: 10.3945/an.113.005025.

15. N. Kalantari et al., "The Association between Dairy Intake, Simple Sugars and Body Mass Index with Expression and Extent of Anger in Female Students," *Iranian Journal of Psychiatry*, vol. 11, no. 1 (January 2016): 43–50, PMID: 27252768.

16. R.A. Stancliffe, T. Thorpe, and M.B. Zemel, "Dairy Attenuates Oxidative and Inflammatory Stress in Metabolic Syndrome," *American Journal of Clinical Nutrition*, vol. 94, no. 2 (August 2011):422–30, doi: 10.3945/ajcn.111.013342.

17. K. Wills, "Your Cheese Addiction Could Be Making You an Emotional Wreck," *New York Post* (August 27, 2018), https://nypost.com/2018/08/27 /your-cheese-addiction-could-be-making-you-an-emotional-wreck.

18. M. Dow, "How to Beat Midlife Brain Fog," DrMikeDow.com (accessed May 1, 2020), https://drmikedow.com/how-to-beat-midlife-brain-fog.

19. K. Brogan, "Two Foods That May Sabotage Your Brain," KellyBroganMD.com (accessed May 6, 2020), https://kellybroganmd.com/two-foods-may -sabotage-brain.

20. J.W. Gerrard, J.S. Richardson, and J. Donat, "Neuropharmacological Evaluation of Movement Disorders That Are Adverse Reactions to Specific Foods," *International Journal of Neuroscience*, vol. 76 (1994): 61–9, doi: 10.3109/00207459408985992.

21. H. Strawbridge, "Going Gluten-free Just Because? Here's What You Need to Know," *Harvard Health Blog* (February 20, 2013), https://www.health .harvard.edu/blog/going-gluten-free-just-because-heres-what-you-need -to-know-201302205916.

22. E. Busby et al., "Mood Disorders and Gluten: It's Not All in Your Mind! A Systematic Review with Meta-Analysis," *Nutrients*, vol. 10, no. 11 (November 2018): 1708, doi: 10.3390/nu10111708.

23. S.E. Milner et al., "Bioactivities of Glycoalkaloids and Their Aglycones from Solanum Species," *Journal of Agricultural and Food Chemistry*, vol. 8, no. 59 (2011): 3454–84, doi: 10.1021/jf200439q.

24. Q. Inam et al., "Effects of Sugar Rich Diet on Brain Serotonin, Hyperphagia and Anxiety in Animal Model of Both Genders," *Pakistan Journal of Pharmaceutical Sciences*, vol. 29, no. 3 (May 2016): 757–63, PMID: 27166525.

25. T.M. Hsu et al., "Effects of Sucrose and High Fructose Corn Syrup Consumption on Spatial Memory Function and Hippocampal Neuroinflammation in Adolescent Rats," *Hippocampus*, vol. 25, no. 2 (2015): 227–39, doi: 10.1002/hipo.22368.

26. K.S. Krabbe et al., "Brain-derived Neurotrophic Factor (BDNF) and Type 2 Diabetes," *Diabetologia*, vol. 50 (February 2007): 431–8, doi: 10.1007/s00125-006-0537-4.

27. N.M. Avena et al., "After Daily Bingeing on a Sucrose Solution, Food Deprivation Induces Anxiety and Accumbens Dopamine/Acetylcholine Imbalance," *Physiology and Behavior*, vol. 94, no. 3 (June 9, 2008): 309–15, doi: 10.1016/j.physbeh.2008.01.008.

28. S.H. Ahmed, K. Guillem, and Y. Vandaele, "Sugar Addiction: Pushing the Drug-Sugar Analogy to the Limit," *Current Opinion in Clinical Nutrition and Metabolic Care*, vol. 16, no. 4 (July 2013): 434–9, doi: 10.1097/MCO.0b013e328361c8b8.

29. Q. Huang et al., "Linking What We Eat to Our Mood: A Review of Diet, Dietary Antioxidants, and Depression," *Antioxidants*, vol. 8, no. 9 (September 5, 2019): 376, doi: 10.3390/antiox8090376.

30. A. Knüppel et al., "Sugar Intake from Sweet Food and Beverages, Common Mental Disorder and Depression: Prospective Findings from the Whitehall II Study," *Scientific Reports*, vol. 7 (July 27, 2017): 6287, doi: 10.1038/s41598-017-05649-7.

31. L.M. Chepulis et al., "The Effects of Long-Term Honey, Sucrose or Sugar-Free Diets on Memory and Anxiety in Rats," *Physiology and Behavior*, vol. 97, nos. 3–4 (June 22, 2009): 359–68, doi: 10.1016/j.physbeh.2009.03.001.

32. G. Koleva, "Binging on Sugar Weakens Memory, UCLA Study Shows," *Forbes* (accessed May 6, 2020), http://www.forbes.com/sites/gerganakoleva/2012/05/17/binging-on-sugar-weakens-memory-ucla-study-shows.

33. A.M. Meyers, D. Mourra, and J.A. Beeler, "High Fructose Corn Syrup Induces Metabolic Dysregulation and Altered Dopamine Signaling in the Absence of Obesity," *PLoS One*, vol. 12, no. 12 (December 29, 2017): e0190206, doi: 10.1371/journal.pone.0190206.

34. Plataforma SINC, "Link Between Fast Food and Depression Confirmed." *ScienceDaily* (March 30, 2012), www.sciencedaily.com/releases/2012/03/120330081352.htm.

35. C.S. Pase et al., "Prolonged Consumption of Trans Fat Favors the Development of Orofacial Dyskinesia and Anxiety-Like Symptoms in Older Rats," *International Journal of Food Sciences and Nutrition*, vol. 65, no. 6 (September 2014): 713–9, doi: 10.3109/09637486.2014.898255.

36. "WHO Plan to Eliminate Industrially-Produced Trans-Fatty Acids from Global Food Supply," World Health Organization (May 14, 2018), https://www.who.int/news-room/detail/14-05-2018-who-plan-to-eliminate-industrially-produced-trans-fatty-acids-from-global-food-supply.

37. A. Sánchez-Villegas et al., "Dietary Fat Intake and the Risk of Depression: The SUN Project," *PLoS One*, vol. 6, no. 1 (January 26, 2011), e16268, doi: 10.1371/journal.pone.0016268.

38. E. Ginter and V. Simko, "New Data on Harmful Effects of Trans-Fatty Acids," *Bratislavské Lekárske Listy*, vol. 117, no. 5 (2016): 251–3, doi: 10.4149/bll_2016_048.

39. M. Hyman, "The Missing Fat You Need to Survive and Thrive," DrMarkHyman.com (accessed May 6, 2020), https://drhyman.com/blog/2016/07/01/the-missing-fat-you-need-to-survive-and-thrive.

40. J.R. Hibbeln, L.R. Nieminen, and W.E. Lands, "Increasing Homicide Rates and Linoleic Acid Consumption among Five Western Countries, 1961–2000," *Lipids*, vol. 39, no. 12 (December 2004): 1207–13, doi: 10.1007/s11745-004-1349-5.

41. M.F. Masana et al., "Dietary Patterns and Their Association with Anxiety Symptoms among Older Adults: The ATTICA Study," *Nutrients*, vol. 11, no. 6 (June 2019): 1250, doi: 10.3390/nu11061250.

42. J.J. DiNicolantonio and J. H. O'Keefe, "Good Fats versus Bad Fats: A Comparison of Fatty Acids in the Promotion of Insulin Resistance, Inflammation, and Obesity," *Missouri Medicine*, vol. 114, no. 4 (July–August 2017): 303–7, PMID: 30228616.

43. A. Samsel and S. Seneff, "Glyphosate, Pathways to Modern Diseases II: Celiac Sprue and Gluten Intolerance," *Interdisciplinary Toxicology*, vol. 6, no. 4 (December 2013): 159–84, doi: 10.2478/intox-2013-0026.

44. World Health Organization, "Constitution of the World Health Organization," in *Basic Documents*, 45th ed., Supplement (October 2006): 1–18, www.who.int/governance/eb/who_constitution_en.pdf.

45. A. K. Choudhary and Y. Y. Lee, "Neurophysiological Symptoms and Aspartame: What Is the Connection?" *Nutritional Neuroscience*, vol. 21 no. 5 (2018): 306–16, doi: 10.1080/1028415X.2017.1288340.

46. M. Briguglio et al., "Dietary Neurotransmitters: A Narrative Review on Current Knowledge," *Nutrients*, vol. 10, no. 5 (May 2018): 521, doi: 10.3390/nu10050591.

47. B. Weiss, "Synthetic Food Colors and Neurobehavioral Hazards: The View from Environmental Health Research," *Environmental Health Perspectives*, vol. 120, no. 1 (January 2012): 1–5, doi: 10.1289/ehp.1103827.

48. C. Graybeal, C. Kiselycznyk, and A. Holmes, "Stress-Induced Deficits in Cognition and Emotionality: A Role for Glutamate," *Current Topics in Behavioral Sciences*, vol. 2012, no. 12 (December 2011): 189–207, doi: 10.1007/7854_2011_193.

49. A. Shimada et al., "Headache and Mechanical Sensitization of Human Pericranial Muscles after Repeated Intake of Monosodium Glutamate (MSG)," *Journal of Headache Pain*, vol. 14, no. 1 (January 2013): 2, doi: 10.1186/1129-2377-14-2.

50. M. Aucoin and S. Bhardwaj, "Generalized Anxiety Disorder and Hypoglycemia Symptoms Improved with Diet Modification," *Case Reports in Psychiatry*, vol. 2016 (2016): 7165425, doi: 10.1155/2016/7165425.

51. U. Naidoo, "Nutritional Strategies to Ease Anxiety," *Harvard Health Blog* (August 29, 2019), https://www.health.harvard.edu/blog/nutritional -strategies-to-ease-anxiety-201604139441.

52. K. Hurley, "Understanding Suicide: From Risk Factors to Prevention, and How to Get Help," Everyday Health (accessed May 6, 2020), https:// www.everydayhealth.com/emotional-health/understanding-suicide -from-risk-factors-prevention-how-get-help.

53. "Beef Jerky and Other Processed Meats Associated with Manic Episodes," Johns Hopkins Medicine Newsroom (July 18, 2018), https://www .hopkinsmedicine.org/news/newsroom/news-releases/beef-jerky -and-other-processed-meats-associated-with-manic-episodes.

54. J. Leech, "Wild vs. Farmed Salmon—Which Type Is Healthier?" *Healthline* (June 4, 2017), https://healthline.com/nutrition/wild-vs-farmed-salmon.

Part II

1. K. Singh, "Nutrient and Stress Management," *Journal of Nutrition and Food Sciences*, vol. 6, no. 4 (June 28, 2016): 528, doi: 10.4172/2155-9600.1000528.

Chapter 6

1. L.M. Kamendulis et al., "Perfluorooctanoic Acid Exposure Triggers Oxidative Stress in the Mouse Pancreas," *Toxicology Reports*, vol. 1 (2014): 513–21, doi: 10.1016/j.toxrep.2014.07.015.

2. A.M. Calafat et al., "Serum Concentrations of 11 Polyfluoroalkyl Compounds in the U.S. Population: Data from the National Health and Nutrition Examination Survey (NHANES) 1999–2000," *Environmental Science and Technology*, vol. 41, no. 7 (2007): 2237–42, doi: 10.1021/es062686m.

3. H.S. Green and S. C. Wang, "First Report on Quality and Purity Evaluations of Avocado Oil Sold in the US," *Food Control*, vol. 116 (October 2020): 107328, doi: 10.1016/j.foodcont.2020.107328.

Chapter 7

1. N. Christie, "3 Key Nutrients for Better Brainpower," Everyday Health (April 8, 2015), https://www.everydayhealth.com/longevity/healthy -eating-recommendations.aspx.

2. X.Z. Sun et al., "Neuroprotective Effects of *Ganoderma lucidum* Polysaccharides Against Oxidative Stress-Induced Neuronal Apoptosis," *Neural Regeneration Research*, vol. 12, no. 6 (June 2017): 953–8, doi: 10.4103/1673-5374.208590.

3. K.K. Vassev et al., "Bee Pollen: Chemical Composition and Therapeutic Application," *Evidence-Based Complementary and Alternative Medicine* : eCAM vol. 2015 (2015): 297425, doi: 10.1155/2015/297425; Erica Cirino, "How Nutritious Is Bee Pollen Exactly?" *Healthline* (June 20, 2017), https://www .healthline.com/health/bee-pollen-benefits#nutrition.

4. T. Clifford et al., "The Potential Benefits of Red Beetroot Supplementation in Health and Disease," *Nutrients*, vol. 7, no. 4 (April 2015): 2801–22, doi: 10.3390/nu7042801.

5. C. Mannuci et al., "Clinical Pharmacology of *Citrus aurantium* and *Citrus sinensis* for the Treatment of Anxiety," *Evidence-Based Complementary and Alternative Medicine*, vol. 2018 (December 2, 2018): 3624094, doi: 10.1155/2018/3624094.

6. F. Que et al., "Advances in Research on the Carrot, an Important Root Vegetable in the Apiaceae Family," *Horticulture Research*, vol. 6 (June 1, 2019): 69, doi: 10.1038/s41438-019-0150-6.

7. A. Nehlig, J.L. Daval, and G. Debry, "Caffeine and the Central Nervous System: Mechanisms of Action, Biochemical, Metabolic and Psychostimulant Effects," *Brain Research. Brain Research Reviews*, vol. 17, no. 2 (1992): 139–70, doi: 10.1016/0165-0173(92)90012-b.

8. M. Brain, C.W. Bryant, and M. Cunningham, "How Caffeine Works," How Stuff Works (accessed April 23, 2020), https://science.howstuffworks.com /caffeine4.htm.

Chapter 8

1. C.N. Sawchuk, "Coping with Anxiety: Can Diet Make a Difference?" Mayo Clinic (May 24, 2017), https://www.mayoclinic.org/diseases-conditions/ generalized-anxiety-disorder/expert-answers/coping-with-anxiety/ faq-20057987.

2. R. Kenny et al., "Effects of Mild Calorie Restriction on Anxiety and Hypothalamic–Pituitary–Adrenal Axis Responses to Stress in the Male Rat," *Physiological Reports*, vol. 2, no. 3 (March 2014): e00265, doi: 10.1002/phy2.265.

3. R. Ullah et al., "Nutritional and Therapeutic Perspectives of Chia (*Salvia hispanica* L.): A Review," *Journal of Food Science and Technology*, vol. 53, no. 4 (April 2016): 1750–8, doi: 10.1007/s13197-015-1967-0.

4. R. Craig and Sons Ltd., "Application for Approval of Whole Chia (*Salvia hispanica* L.) Seed and Ground Whole Seed as Novel Food Ingredient," Food Standard Agency, U.K. Commission Decision 2009/827/EC, Company Representative Mr. D. Armstrong, Northern Ireland, 2004.

5. U.S. Department of Health and Human Services and U.S. Department of Agriculture, *Dietary Guidelines for Americans 2015–2020*, Eighth Edition (December 2015), https://www.dietaryguidelines.gov/current-dietary-guidelines/2015-2020-dietary-guidelines.

6. J.C. King and J.L. Slavin, "White Potatoes, Human Health, and Dietary Guidance," *Advances in Nutrition*, vol. 4, no. 3 (May 6, 2013): S393–401, doi: 10.3945/an.112.003525.

Chapter 10

1. A. Hirose et al., "Tomato Juice Intake Increases Resting Energy Expenditure and Improves Hypertriglyceridemia in Middle-Aged Women: An Open-Label, Single-Arm Study," *Nutrition Journal*, vol. 14 (2015): 34, doi: 10.1186/s12937-015-0021-4.

2. S. Argawal and A. V. Rao, "Tomato Lycopene and Its Role in Human Health and Chronic Diseases," *CMAJ*, vol. 163, no. 6 (September 19, 2000): 739–44. PMCID: PMC80172.

3. K. Ganesan and B. Xu, "Polyphenol-Rich Lentils and Their Health Promoting Effects," *International Journal of Molecular Sciences*, vol. 18, no. 11 (November 10, 2017): 2390, doi: 10.3390/ijms18112390.

4. C. Northrup, "How to Keep Your Breasts Healthy for Life," *Christiane Northrup M.D.* blog (accessed August 8, 2018), https://www.drnorthrup.com/breast-cancer-keep-breasts-healthy-cancer-free.

5. A. Hosseini et al., "Hypnotic Effect of Red Cabbage (*Brassica oleracea*) on Pentobarbital-Induced Sleep in Mice," *Journal of Pharmacy and BioAllied Sciences*, vol. 10, no. 1 (January–March 2018): 48–53, doi: 10.4103/jpbs.JPBS_215_17.

Chapter 11

1. S.N. Young, "How to Increase Serotonin in the Human Brain Without Drugs," *Journal of Psychiatry and Neuroscience*, vol. 32, no. 6 (November 2007): 394–9, PMID: 18043762.

2. T.C. Wallace, R. Murray, and K.M. Zelman, "The Nutritional Value and Health Benefits of Chickpeas and Hummus," *Nutrients*, vol. 8, no. 12 (December 2016): 766, doi: 10.3390/nu8120766.

3. A.L.G. Júnior et al., "Anxiolytic Effect of Anacardic Acids from Cashew (*Anacardium occidentale*) Nut Shell in Mice," *IUBMB Life*, vol. 70, no. 5 (2018): 420–31, doi: 10.1002/iub.1738.

Chapter 12

1. D. Średnicka-Tober et al., "Composition Differences Between Organic and Conventional Meat: A Systematic Literature Review and Meta-Analysis," *British Journal of Nutrition*, vol. 115, no. 6 (March 28, 2016): 994–1011, doi: 10.1017/S0007114515005073.

2. F. Haghighatdoost and B.M. Nobakht, "Effect of Conjugated Linoleic Acid on Blood Inflammatory Markers: A Systematic Review and Meta-Analysis on Randomized Controlled Trials," *European Journal of Clinical Nutrition*, vol. 72, no. 8 (August 2018): 1071–82, doi: 10.1038/s41430-017-0048-z.

3. "The Burning Question: Do I Need to Buy Organic Chicken?" *Health* (April 27, 2011), https://www.health.com/nutrition/the-burning-question -do-i-need-to-buy-organic-chicken.

4. Ibid.

5. U.J. Yang, T.S. Park, and S.M. Shim, "Protective Effect of Chlorophyllin and Lycopene from Water Spinach Extract on Cytotoxicity and Oxidative Stress Induced by Heavy Metals in Human Hepatoma Cells," *Journal of Toxicology and Environmental Health*, vol. 76, no. 23 (2013): 1307–15, doi: 10.1080/15287394.2013.851632.

6. A.V. Ferlemi et al., "Rosemary Tea Consumption Results to Anxiolytic- and Anti-Depressant-Like Behavior of Adult Male Mice and Inhibits All Cerebral Area and Liver Cholinesterase Activity; Phytochemical Investigation and in Silico Studies," *Chemico-Biological Interactions*, vol. 237 (July 25, 2015): 47–57, doi: 10.1016/j.cbi.2015.04.013.

7. P. Nematolahi et al., "Effects of *Rosmarinus officinalis* L. on Memory Performance, Anxiety, Depression, and Sleep Quality in University Students: A Randomized Clinical Trial," *Complementary Therapies in Clinical Practice*, vol. 30 (February 2018): 24–8, doi: 10.1016/j.ctcp.2017.11.004.

8. W. Sayorwan et al., "Effects of Inhaled Rosemary Oil on Subjective Feelings and Activities of the Nervous System," *Scientia Pharmaceutica*, vol. 81, no. 2 (April–June 2018): 531–42, doi: 10.3797/scipharm.1209-05.

9. P.R. Cheeke, S. Piacente, and W. Oleszek, "Anti-Inflammatory and Anti-Arthritic Effects of Yucca Schidigera: A Review," *Journal of Inflammation*, vol. 3 (March 29, 2006): 6, doi: 10.1186/1476-9255-3-6.

Chapter 13

1. "A Good Guide to Good Carbs: The Glycemic Index," *Healthbeat*, Harvard Medical School (accessed April 21, 2020), https://www.health.harvard.edu/healthbeat/a-good-guide-to-good-carbs-the-glycemic-index.

2. A.N. Gearhardt et al., "Neural Correlates of Food Addiction," *Archives of General Psychiatry*, vol. 68, no. 8 (2011): 808–16, doi: 10.1001/archgenpsychiatry.2011.32.

3. A.L.G. Júnior et al., "Anxiolytic Effect of Anacardic Acids from Cashew (*Anacardium occidentale*) Nut Shell in Mice," *IUBMB Life*, vol. 70, no. 5 (2018): 420–31, doi: 10.1002/iub.1738.

4. R.D. Damavandi et al., "Effects of Daily Consumption of Cashews on Oxidative Stress and Atherogenic Indices in Patients with Type 2 Diabetes: A Randomized, Controlled-Feeding Trial," *International Journal of Endocrinology & Metabolism*, vol. 17, no. 1 (January 2019): e70744, doi: 10.5812/ijem.70744.

5. L. Stojanovskaet et al., "Maca Reduces Blood Pressure and Depression, in a Pilot Study in Postmenopausal Women," *Climacteric*, vol. 18, no. 1 (February 2015): 68–79, doi: 10.3109/13697137.2014.929649.

INDEX

INDEX OF RECIPES
AND INGREDIENTS

ACKNOWLEDGMENTS

I am incredibly grateful for the opportunity to write about this subject matter, of food relating to mental health such as anxiety.

Thank you to my publishing team at Hay House: Patty Gift, vice president, editorial, for the encouragement to write this new book; Reid Tracy, president and CEO, for consistent support; Nicolette Salamanca Young, editor, so happy to work on another project with you—we are on a roll!; Anne Barthel, go New York team, woo-hoo!; and Lindsay McGinty, associate director, publicity and book marketing. I am so grateful for all those at work behind the scenes who contributed to this book—thank you so much. I hope you know the extent of my gratitude and recognize how many people are being healed because of your contribution of talent, skill, effort, and energy. I value the teamwork.

Thank you to my developmental editor, Stephanie Gunning. This is the first book we couldn't sit side by side (because of COVID-19 distancing) and drink green juice and eat chocolate balls together! But we still ate our brain foods while putting the manuscript together—only apart this time.

Thank you, Dr. Rashid Buttar, for all the incredible work you do in the world! The more brains we can protect, educate, and help, the better. Thank you, Dr. Ashton, for offering your expertise as a naturopathic doctor. Thank you to Dr. Mark Hyman, Dr. Christiane Northrup, Dr. Josh Axe, Jim Kiwk, Max Lugavere, Vani Hari, and other wonderful friends and influential, dedicated health leaders for endorsing this book.

Thank you to my family for your unconditional love and support: my Aunty Tammy, my rock; my Uncle Michael; and my cousin Bernie. To my sisters, Nadine, Caitlin, and Lauren, I love you more than you will ever truly know. To my mum for constantly inspiring me forward. I love you, Nanna and Laurie. I am also grateful to my extended family: to Sav, to Steven, to Rock, and especially to Carol

Lucas—you alone have provided me a solid foundation upon which I was able to grow—thank you so very much.

Thank you, Monica Rowsom, for your unbelievable generosity in helping me with this project . . . and life! Thank you, Peter Rowsom and Alexander, Cali—and you too, Skipper. Looking forward to enjoying more healthy recipes with you guys.

Thank you to my beautiful friends for your support and grace. Gloria Pope and Bill, my quaranteam! Gloria, I have loved doing isolated workouts with you in Central Park, home workouts, enjoying fine meals, and, of course, superfood smoothies during the writing of this book.

Thank you, Sahara Rose and Cassandra Bodzak, for the profound birthday prayer when I turned 33 while writing this book and for helping me set the intention of this year. Maria Marlowe, I would have been writing part of this book in Dubai had your wedding travel not stopped because of COVID. Jill de Jong, I am so grateful for your beautiful, energizing, fun, adventurous spirit in my life. Natalie Jill, I am so grateful to know you, you unstoppable, gorgeous woman—I think of you every time I make the SunButter Cups. Thank you to the Rockstar IG group: Abbey Gibb, Amber Lilyestrom, Cayla Craft, Christine Hassler, Christine Olivia, Danny J, Allyson Byrd, Keri Glassman, Brooke Thomas, Liz German, Sarah Fontenot, and Sarah Pendrick, I love our female empowerment social media group! Alyson Charles, you are such a rock star soul! Tara Mackey, sis, thank you for being you. Sarah Stewart, you are an angel.

Thank you, Caroline Tarnofsky and Alexandra Strimbu, for holding down the Earth Diet fort while I was writing this book, and thank you for keeping the business going and growing. Thank you as well, Ellie Simms, for your beautiful spirit. You are all truly earth angels contributing to helping others find health and healing.

Thank you, Dr. Daniel Fenster, for your friendship and support. Thank you so much for giving me a platform to coach people one-on-one at Complete Wellness NYC. The most fulfilling thing I could ever do on a Thursday in New York City is work with you and the team! Thank you, Jan Fenster, for your breathing techniques and essential oils—you are such an angel in how you calm everyone down and we can somehow all breathe so much better in your presence. Thank you, Dr. Dana Cohen, for your support and guidance. You are amazing and I am aware how very privileged I am to be able to have worked with you for three years. Thank you, Dr. Kay, for telling me to keep going with this mission, even when it looked like rough seas ahead. Thank you for all your good ideas! And thank you to the rest of the Complete Wellness NYC team. Yossie, I am grateful to you for keeping it all together. Stephanie Urena, thank you for keeping the front on point—love seeing your beautiful face every workday! Jeanette, I am grateful to you for keeping the back together. Thank you, Dr. H., for helping keep my body in check with acupuncture and cupping. Thank you, Peter Nesi and Liz Correale, for holding us all together during quarantine. Thank you also to the patients at CW; I love working with you and seeing you heal and transform your lives one step at a time. This makes me the happiest.

Thank you, Heather Dean, for teaching me tools to get control over my mind. I hope to someday be able to tell people about your book, once it's written!

Thank you to the SunButter team! SunButter has changed my life—literally; it's changed the evolution of my recipes, and you can see by all the recipes in this book that include your product as an ingredient how much it has impacted my health and the lives of so many. Thank you to a brilliant team and friends, Justin LaGosh, Geri Tollefson, Wyatt Mund, Jayden Howie, Kim Graw, and Nadine Doetterl.

Thank you to the Nutiva team! I fueled my brain greatly during writing this book with the coconut oil, MCT oil, hempseeds, chia seeds, plant protein, MCT powder, avocado oil, vegan ghee, and, of course, yes, you guessed it . . . your incredible, buttery-tasting coconut oil! Wow, I am just realizing how much of my kitchen cabinet and fridge is made up of your products. My brain owes part of its life fuel, and some of the creation of this book, to foods your company manufactures! Thank you for providing such epic, life-giving foods to so many people, world changers Steve

Naccarato, Prapti Rana, Madalyn Crum, Chris Amsler, Yulanda Smith, Alessandra Vejby, and Virginia Watkins. John Roulac, the OG, thank you for inspiring me and the world! You are a legend who pioneered coconut oil and hemp in the United States.

Thank you to the Vitacost team. Our partnership is going on eight years now! It is a genuine pleasure working with you and I am so grateful that you make organic living much more affordable for me and millions of others! Thank you, Katie Kaleita, Rebecca Chopin, Guy Burgstahler, Katie Burger, Thomas Cary, and Terri Smith.

Thank you to the Explore Cuisine team! I love that my diet can now safely include pasta once again! Thank you for making such gluten-free deliciousness, Greg Forbes, Joe Spronz, Jim Magner, Elizabeth Tashiro, Alex Pegon, Christine Grieco, Silvia Graf, Per Nilson, and Brooke Vaccarella. Once we can travel again, I am so excited to see the Explore Cuisine pasta factory in Italy!

Thank you to the Sawtooth team. Yours is such a forward-thinking marketing agency—and more. Thank you, Kristi Bridges, Jackie Finger, Mike, Lisa Paccagnini, and Alana Roolaart. I love working with you guys and coming up with creative ways to spread the good news about healthy foods to mainstream media!

Thank you to the Hu Kitchen team: Jordan Brown, Jessica Brown Karp, and Gabby Bellettieri. You *would* believe me when I said how much Hu chocolate I ate during the writing of this book in the midst of New York City's social distancing lockdown. Well, you saw it all on my IG stories! Thank you, guys, for making healthier chocolate accessible to everyone in the United States; it's contributing to the health of so many people's brains!

Thank you to Ancient Nutrition; I am honored to be an Ancient pioneer.

Thank you to the Juice Press team! I was able to enjoy cold-pressed juices while writing this book during COVID-19 because of delivery. If any juice bar knows how to be adaptable with the times, it is yours! Thank you, Daniel Ceballos, Marcus Antebi, and Michael Karsch. Without Juice Press, I wouldn't have the time to drink as many vegetable juices.

Thank you, Doug Evans, for your support and sprout wisdom!

Thank you, Mae Rose, for helping me to detoxify my body when I was at a physical rock bottom and helping me get my life back on track. Thank you, Craig and Steph Green, for your prayers and the OG yogis and juicers! Also, thank you, JD, Shawn, and Shane Chapman.

Thank you to my awesome friends Roxxe Ireland, Inna Mel, Heidi Williams, Kristy Rao, Alie and Justin Mitchell, Melissa Mitchell, Max Goldberg, Steph and Josh Tarnofsky. Jae Bae, you get a shout-out too, cos just thinking of your face makes me smile so good. Brenda Vongova and Sarah Deanna, my other sis. Love you guys!

Thank you to Summer Rose, my quarantine neighbor. I loved all our iso-dancing! And thank you for filming my recipe videos during lockdown. Thank you, also, for your professional organization and decluttering of my room and apartment. Now that I have a clearer space, I can think so much better because I always have a fresh space in which to work. Wow, what a difference you have made to my life, my home, and my creative process.

Thank you, Mary Mucci! I have loved doing all our Long Island Naturally segments on News 12 over the years! It's always so fun to work with you!

Thank you for existing in this work, Dr. Jess Peatross, and for being the voice you are. Your courage is so admirable. You are a dream-come-true kind of doctor!

Thank you, Bec Donlan (aka Sweat with Bec) for the Booty Band workouts and keeping my blood flowing while sitting down so much to write this book.

Theo Quinto, you are a legend! Thank you, Sovereign Silver team.

Special thanks to my publicity team, Adam Weiss and Angela Gorman.

Robert Scott Bell, Nancy, Elijah, and Ariana, thank you for your support and fun times over the years; you, Bell family, are amazing! You have a special place in my heart. Let's go to the snow again soon, please!

Special thanks also belong to Daryl Gioffre. Your energy and work are so needed and appreciated in this world.

Ty and Charlene Bollinger, thank you so much for all your support, wisdom, and kindness over the years. Thank you for providing me and other health advocates with a platform to reach so many people. I hope you get the magnitude of what you have done for the world and in people's lives and health.

Thank you to bright lights Sarah Stewart and Craig Clemens! You guys are beyond epic. Thank you for your friendship, love, and support, and for creating the Rising Glen community.

Thank you, Mike Dow, for all your love and support. You are such a positive force in the world. I love sharing healthy brain recipes for your books, too. *The Brain Fog Solution* is what's up!

Scott Prentiss, thank you for all your guidance, support, and genius ingredient-combining ideas. I am excited for all the sweet things ahead!

Thank you, Tamara Martucci and Molly Lukins Burke. Your company Food and Mood is helping New Yorkers and beyond with mindful eating, especially in a corporate structure. Love you, boss babes.

Thank you to Suzie and Vinny Lobdell and the rest of the Intellipure team. Thank you for bringing the finest air-quality technology to the world. I felt so safe and comfortable working from my apartment with purified air during a pandemic and writing this book. It has made a profound difference on my lungs, breathing, brain, and overall health.

Thank you, Howard Hoffman, Christina, and Paul Lepore. You would all probably believe me when I said how much pHresh Greens and cacao powder I consumed during the writing of this book.

Thank you, Joyce Meyer, for sharing your wisdom with me and the world. Your teachings have helped me to heal my soul and become a better everything.

Thank you, Geney Kim, for all your love and support. Special thanks to Shane Hofer. Hope to see you guys at a food event soon!

Thank you to my sisters in Christ and our Bible Study Babes group. All the walks in Palm Beach, prayers, Pilates, and biblical wisdom helped me finish this book with confidence. Thank you: Ginelle Ruffa, Giana Ruffa, Izabela Sederowska, Cassie Mae, Keeley, Sommer, Tea, Sabrina, Keri, Emily, Krista, Sarah, Katie, and Elizabeth. Thank you, Mama G, for your pharmaceutical expertise and you just being you!

Thank you, Sherri Tenpenny, for being a fearless leader.

Thank you, Patricia Bragg, for inspiring me to continue on with being a WOO-HOO person. Thank you, Lesley Zahara and the OG Bragg team! Thank you for bringing apple cider vinegar, amino acids, and so much health and healing to the world. Your legacy will live on in the world and the universe forever.

Thank you, Joyce Walker Robertson, for the mostly heavenly organic bed; I had the best nights' sleep—ever—while writing this book.

Thank you to all the health coaches and nutritionists that I haven't met yet, for having the heart and passion and helping so many others. Don't give up, it's a commendable mission you are on, and the world needs you!

I am forever grateful for the presence of the late Wayne Dyer and Louise Hay in my life and the growth that they initiated in me. The interview I did with Wayne on his radio show is my favorite interview to date. I remember eating three chocolate balls beforehand to calm my nerves. A special thank-you also goes to Diane Ray DePasquale. You had a profound impact on my online-air work; I am incredibly grateful for you.

Thank you, David Fulcher. I am next-level excited about our Anxiety-Free supplements and how many people they can help. Thank you to the Forsyth team, John, Jonathon, and Sonja, for putting together the most effective and great-quality supplements with us!

Thank you, Javi Ergas, the best roomie I could ask for! Our late-night talks and adventures to Westerly Market were refreshing during this book process.

Thank you to everyone I may be forgetting who has influenced my thinking in any way that has contributed to this book from the time I began writing to the time it was launched. You know who you are. My thank-you pages are always so long, but I get a lot of help and support so I want to acknowledge everything people are giving to me that keeps me going.

I thank God for the beautiful work that has been done in my life, which is endless. I am in awe, wonder, and gratitude every day, wondering what You will do next. Thank You for the lessons and for teaching me how I can be of better service to others. Thank You for showing me how food can heal.

Is it weird also to thank myself? Because I want to thank myself for showing up, not giving up, and being relentless in finding a way to heal. No matter what happens in my life, I've made a commitment to get back up again and again when I get knocked down. I will continue to stand tall even through the roughest periods of depression and anxiety.

And lastly, thank YOU, dear reader. If you have ever thought something positive for me, prayed for me, or told one of your loved ones about my books or healing recipes, please know that I am sending you great energy right now! This world can be brutally rough, so I am thankful for even a little bit of your love!

ABOUT THE AUTHOR

Liana Werner-Gray is a certified nutritionist and natural food and healing chef. She is a passionate advocate for healthy diet and lifestyle, and author of three best-selling books about wholesome nutrition: *Cancer-Free with Food*, *The Earth Diet*, and *10-Minute Recipes*. Liana is the resident health and nutrition coach at Complete Wellness NYC. Since 2009, she has been lecturing and teaching internationally about the benefits of consuming natural, whole food and visiting schools, corporations, churches, libraries, and police departments to educate people on making healthier choices.

Liana and her work have been featured on NBC, ABC News, CBS, and Fox television networks; on *The Wendy Williams Show*, and News 12 NY, among other programs; on iHeart Radio and WABC radio; in print publications including *Woman's Own* and *The Sun* (U.K.); and in lifestyle blogs such as *Yahoo Beauty*, *Bustle*, and *Pop Sugar*. She has contributed articles to Mindbodygreen, Huffington Post, Food Matters, and Heal Your Life. As a speaker, she has presented at online events including the Keto Edge Summit and TEDx Orient; and she has appeared onstage at the I Can Do It! Conference and the Truth About Cancer Live.

Liana was born in Perth, Australia, raised in Alice Springs and Arno Bay, and now resides in New York City. Visit her at LianaWernerGray.com.

Hay House Titles of Related Interest

YOU CAN HEAL YOUR LIFE, the movie,
starring Louise Hay & Friends
(available as a 1-DVD program, an expanded 2-DVD set,
and an online streaming video)
Learn more at www.hayhouse.com/louise-movie

THE SHIFT, the movie,
starring Dr. Wayne W. Dyer
(available as a 1-DVD program, an expanded 2-DVD set,
and an online streaming video)
Learn more at www.hayhouse.com/the-shift-movie

***

Eliminating Stress, Finding Inner Peace,
by Brian L. Weiss, M.D.

*Feeding You Lies: How to Unravel the Food Industry's
Playbook and Reclaim Your Health,* by Vani Hari

*Heal Your Drained Brain: Naturally Relieve Anxiety,
Combat Insomnia, and Balance Your Brain in Just 14 Days,*
by Dr. Mike Dow

*A Little Peace of Mind: The Revolutionary Solution
for Freedom from Anxiety, Panic Attacks and Stress,* by Nicola Bird

*The Tapping Solution for Manifesting
Your Greatest Self,* by Nick Ortner

All of the above are available at your local bookstore,
or may be ordered by contacting Hay House (see next page).

***

Listen. Learn. Transform.

Listen to the audio version
of this book for FREE!

Unlock endless wisdom, fresh perspectives, and life-changing tools from world-renowned authors and teachers—helping you embrace vibrant health in your body, mind, and spirit. With the *Hay House Unlimited* Audio app, you can learn and grow in a way that fits your lifestyle . . . and your daily schedule.

With your membership, you can:

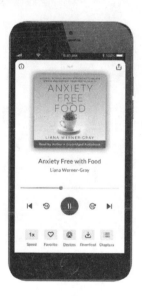

- Develop a healthier mind, body, and spirit through natural remedies, healthy foods, and powerful healing practices.

- Explore thousands of audiobooks, meditations, immersive learning programs, podcasts, and more.

- Access exclusive audios you won't find anywhere else.

- Experience completely unlimited listening. No credits. No limits. No kidding.

Try for FREE!

Visit **hayhouse.com/try-free** to start your free trial and get one step closer to living your best life.

A powerful blend of Ashwaganda, Spirulina, Turmeric, Flax Oil, Chlorella, Schisandra, and more!

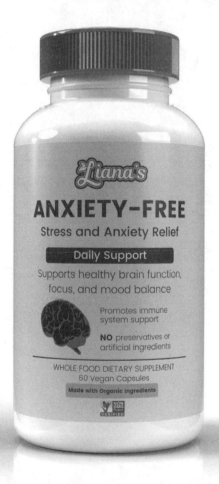